INSULIN RESISTANCE DIET

THE COMPLETE GUIDE TO PREVENT DIABETES WITH LOW SUGAR AND LOW GI RECIPES

SOFIA FOSTER

Table of Contents

PART 1

PART 1.1:

INSULIN RESISTANCE DIET

INTRODUCTION

If you find you are being warned by your doctor that you are at high risk of developing diabetes, or that you have insulin resistance, you're not alone. In fact, it's believed that the number of diabetics is going to double from around 190 million to 325 million within the next couple of decades. A study performed in 2002 found that 32.2% of the population in the US are insulin resistant.

Knowing how insulin resistance works on a cellular level helps people know the best ways to treat and prevent type 2 diabetes. Individuals who suffer from diabetes mellitus and obese people are often insulin resistant. Many studies have discovered that an insulin resistance diet and exercise can alter the pathways and slow down the onset of insulin resistance.

It's safe to say that if we look at ways to change our habits, and pay attention to what we do, we can make some improvements to our life. An insulin resistance diet can help you to lose weight and will turn regulate your blood glucose and insulin levels so that your chances of developing diabetes are lowered.

It's possible that insulin resistance is the leading cause of many of today's chronic diseases. These diseases are collectively killing over a million people each year. The good thing is that it can easily be improved with some simple changed in your eating, lifestyle, and exercise habits. Preventing the chance of insulin resistance is probably the best thing you can do to make sure you live a long, healthy life.

There are plenty of books on this subject on the market, thanks again for choosing this one! Every effort was made to ensure it is full of as much useful information as possible. Please enjoy!

Congratulations on downloading your personal copy of *Insulin Resistance Diet Plan for Type 2 Diabetics*. Thank you for doing so.

UNDERSTAND THE RESISTANCE

There are times when our cells quit responding to our insulin. When this happens, you are likely suffering from insulin resistance. Your cells become resistant to insulin. When your body becomes resistant, your pancreas will respond by producing more insulin to try and reduce your blood sugar levels. When this happens you develop hyperinsulinemia, which is when the blood contains high levels of insulin. Let's make this a little easier, let's look at the separate parts of insulin resistance.

Metabolism

Metabolism is probably one of the most misunderstood processes that the body goes through. Your metabolism works as a collection of chemical reactions that happens in your cells to help you convert food into energy. As you are reading this, a thousand metabolic reactions are happening. There are two main metabolic channels.

- Catabolism is the process your body goes through when breaking down you food components, as in fats, proteins, and carbs, into simpler parts, which are then used for energy. To better understand it, look at it as if it is your destructive metabolism. Your cells break down fats and carbs to release their energy; this ensures that your body can fuel an anabolic reaction.
- Anabolism is the contrastive metabolism which works to build and store energy. When your cells perform an anabolic process, it helps to grow new cells and to maintain your body tissues, and it also helps to store energy that you can use later.

The nervous and hormone systems control these processes. When you look at how many calories you should consume in a day, you have to check your body's total energy expenditure. What you eat, how much you move, how you rest, and how well your tissues and cells recuperate will all go into figuring out your total energy expenditure.

Your metabolism is made up of three main components:

1. Basal metabolic rate – this how many calories you body can burn while at rest, and also contributes to 50 to 80 percent of the amount of energy you body uses.

2. How much energy is used during activity – this is how many calories your body burns when you are active. This takes up 20% of your total expenditure.

3. Warming effects of your food – this is how many calories you use when you eat, digest, and metabolize your food.

Insulin

Insulin is a hormone that the pancreas produces and releases into your blood. Insulin helps to keep your blood sugar at a reasonable level by promoting cell growth and division, protein and lipid metabolism, regulating carbohydrates, and glucose uptake. Insulin helps your cells absorb glucose to use for energy.

After you eat, and your blood sugar levels rise, insulin is released. The glucose and insulin travel throughout your blood to your cells. It helps to stimulate the muscle tissue and liver; helps liver, fat, and muscle cells to absorb glucose; and lowers glucose levels by reducing the glucose production in your liver.

People who suffer from type 1 or type 2 diabetes may have to take insulin shot to help their bodies metabolize glucose correctly. Type 1 diabetic's pancreas doesn't make insulin, and the beta cells have been destroyed. There's typically no chance of preventing type 1, and most of the time a person is born with it. Type 2 diabetic's pancreas still makes insulin, but the body doesn't respond to it.

Symptoms

If you go to the doctor, they will likely test your fasting insulin levels. If you have high levels, then chances are you are insulin resistant. You can also do an oral glucose tolerance test. This is where you will be given a dose of glucose, and they will check your blood sugar levels for the next few hours.

People who are obese or overweight, and people with a lot of fat in the mid-section, are at a greater risk of being insulin resistant. Acanthosis nigrans, a skin condition characterized by dark spots on the skin, can be a symptom of insulin resistance. Also, if you have low HDL and high triglycerides, then your chances are higher as well.

For the most part, insulin resistance and pre-diabetes have no significant symptoms. They main way to find out if you have either one is to get tested by your doctor. Now, you're probably wondering how to know if you should be tested. Here are some reasons why you should:

- Body Mass Index over 25
- Over age 45
- Have CVD
- Physically inactive
- Parent or sibling with diabetes
- Family background of Pacific Islander American, Hispanic/Latino, Asian American, Native American, Alaska Native, or African American
- Had a baby that weighed more than 9 pounds
- Diagnoses of gestational diabetes
- High blood pressure – 140/90 or higher
- HDL below 35 or triglyceride above 250
- Have polycystic ovary syndrome

If your tests come back as normal, be sure to be retested every three years, at least. But, you don't have to wait until you get positive test results to start changing your life. In fact, if you have any of the risk factors, even if it's just a family history, you start changing now, and you may never have to hear that diagnoses.

INSULIN RESISTANCE DIET

Years of research has found that excess weight is the primary cause of insulin resistance. This means that weight loss can help your body better respond to insulin. Studies performed by the Diabetes Prevention Program have found that people who are pre-diabetic and insulin resistance can prevent or slow down the development of diabetes by fixing their diet.

Guidelines

Here are the main seven ways you go start to develop an insulin resistance diet:

1.   Reduce Carbohydrate Intake

Studies that have been published in *Diabetes, Metabolic Syndrome and Obesity* suggest that controlling the number of carbohydrates you eat is essential in controlling your glycemic index. You can count all carbs you eat, but it's best if you make sure you consume your carbs from dairy products, legumes, whole grains, fruits, and veggies.

2.   Stay Away From Sweetened Beverages

All sugars will raise your blood sugar levels, but the American Diabetes Association has now advised, specifically, to avoid sugar-sweetened drinks. This includes iced tea, fruit drinks, soft drinks, and vitamin or energy water drinks that have artificial sweeteners, concentrates, high fructose corn syrup, or sucrose.

3. Consume More Fiber

Glycemia is improved in people who consume more than 50 grams of fiber each day. Large prospective cohort studies have shown that whole grain consumption is associated with a lower risk of type 2 diabetes.

4. Consume Healthy Fats

Studies have shown that fatty acids are more important than total fat. People who suffer from insulin resistance should consume unsaturated fats instead of trans fatty acids or saturated fats.

5. Consume Plenty of Protein

International Journal of Vitamin and Nutrition Research published a study in 2011 that discovered people who were on a diet to treat obesity had better results when they consumed more protein.

6. Consume Dairy

More and more studies are finding that dairy consumption is linked to a reduced risk of type 2 diabetes.

7. Watch Your Portions

Losing weight is key in reducing your risk for diabetes. One great way to do that controls your portion sizes. It's best to eat more small meals instead of three large meals.

Bad Foods

When you start the insulin resistance diet, there are certain foods that you need to avoid, or at least reduce your intake of. Here are some of the foods that you need to watch out for.

- Red meat – contains lots of saturated fats that can exacerbate the problems

- Certain cheeses – cheese that is high in fat will cause more problems

- Fried food – this is a bad dietary choice no matter what diet you're on

- Grains – processed or refined carbs can lead higher insulin levels

- Potatoes – these foods turn into sugar in your system

- Pumpkin – these are just like potatoes

- Carrots – these aren't entirely bad for you, just limit your intake because they are high in sugar

- Doughnuts – these are full insulin raising ingredients

- Alcohol – these turn straight to sugar when you drink them

Good Foods

Now that you know the main foods you should stay away from, here are the foods you should consume.

- Broccoli, Spinach, Collard greens – these, as well as most other leafy greens, are a great source of magnesium, zinc, vitamin E, C, and A
- Broccoli sprouts
- Swiss Chard, Romaine Lettuce, Arugula, Green Cabbage, and Kale – these also contain high amounts of nutrients
- Blueberries – contain anthocyanins which simulate the release of adiponectin which helps regular blood sugar
- Indian gooseberry – these can regulate blood sugar and reduce hyperglycemia
- Walnuts – any nut is great food for an insulin resistance diet

These are just a few of some of the foods you should consume. Many other foods have the same properties as the ones on this list, as well as a few other types of benefits.

LONG-TERM MANAGEMENT

Once you have started a diet, the hardest thing is sticking with it. The good thing about this diet is that it isn't anything drastic, and you can quickly change your diet with a few tweaks. To ensure that you have lasting results, let's look at some of the best ways to maintain.

Be sure to keep up regular exercise. Exercise can help lower your blood sugar, reduce body fat, and help you lose weight. Your cells will also become more insulin sensitive as well. You don't have to do anything spectacular either. Any movement will help you; gardening, running, swimming, walking, or dancing all count for exercise.

Remember that weight loss isn't going to be linear. You may start dropping pounds when you first start, but you will eventually hit a plateau. You have to be proactive with your diet. When you notice you are hitting a plateau, start to make little changes to push past it.

Try to pay attention to when you eat. If you notice that you eat when you are stress, upset, sad, bored, lonely, or low on energy take note of it. Look for other ways to move past those emotions to prevent emotional eating.

Find some cheerleaders. I don't mean paying people to follow you around all day cheering, that would get annoying. I mean you should find a support system. The main reason why diet programs like Jenny Craig and Weight

Watchers works are because of the meeting and people to talk to. There's no need to pay big bucks for this thought. You can get your family and friends to help you out, and you can probably find a Facebook group to help you out.

Side Effects

With any diet, you will experience some side effects. These side effects will either be longer-term or short-term. Let's look at some side effects that you may experience when you begin the insulin resistance diet.

- Short-term:
  - Cravings – this is normal when you start to change your diet. Your body becomes freaked out when you start to eat healthier foods and reduce the snack foods that you're used to eating. Keep reminding yourself why you're doing this. The cravings will eventually pass.
  - Headaches – this is because your body has become addicted to the processed foods you're used to eating. You're going to withdrawals. Once you get all the bad food out of your system, the headaches will stop.
  - Lower energy – this is another symptom you will have because of withdrawals. Your energy levels will drop. Your

body is doing a lot of work when you start eating healthier, so be patient with it.

- Long-term:
  - Weight loss – this is probably the best thing that will happen to you on this diet. Weight loss will help to improve all of your health problems.
  - Less hunger and cravings – you may start out having more cravings, but once that phase passes, you won't be bothered with the hunger and cravings like you used to be.
  - Lower blood pressure – a diet that is low in sugar and trans and saturated fats, your blood pressure will lower. This reduces your risk of heart disease, heart attack, stroke, and several other health problems.
  - More energy – getting rid of high glycemic index foods will give bursts of energy that you have never had. Plus, you will no longer have the rollercoaster effect from your blood sugar highs and lows.
  - Better mood and concentration – with your old diet, you probably had mood boosts followed by a sudden plummet. With the insulin resistance diet, you will keep a more steady mood and concentration throughout the day.

- o   Better immune system – since you won't be consuming as many inflammatory and allergenic foods you will be able to improve your overall immune system and health.

- o   Increased digestion – with this diet you will reduce your intake of sugar, dairy, and gluten. These foods are the most common foods to cause digestive problems. Since you won't be consuming as many of these foods, your digestive system will work better. You will also increase your fiber intake, so this will aid your gastrointestinal tract as well.

As you can see, the long-term side effects are better than the short-term side effects; there are also more long-term effects. It's easy to see the good outweighs the bad. It's a no brainer that this is an easy and simple diet to follow.

DIET PLAN

To help get you started, here is a 5-day meal plan. All of the recipes will follow in the next chapter.

Day One

Breakfast: Basil and Tomato Frittata

Frittatas are the perfect breakfast to help use up leftovers. Pair this with a slice of whole grain toast and fruit.

Lunch: Carrot and Butternut Squash Soup

You'll never go back to canned soups after you try this.

Dinner: Grilled Shrimp Skewers

This is a quick meal because shrimp only takes a few minutes to cook.

Day Two

Breakfast: Pecan, Carrot, and Banana Muffins

This is a meal you can serve to your friends, and nobody will ever know that they are healthy. It's the perfect guilt-free treat.

Lunch: Lemony Hummus

Creating your hummus is a great meal. You have control over its flavor and salt levels.

Dinner: Chicken Tortilla Soup

This is perfect if you have some leftover chicken. This spicy soup will satisfy everyone.

Day Three

Breakfast: Dried Fruit, Seeds, and Nuts Granola

This is great to mix up a large amount on the weekend and portion it out for the following week.

There is a high carb content because of the dried fruit, but you can easily fix that by reducing the fruit or leaving it out entirely.

Lunch: Quinoa Tabbouleh Salad

Quinoa is the perfect food because not only is it gluten-free, but it's also considered a protein. This is a delicious meal for meat-eaters and vegetarians.

Dinner: Rice and Beef Stuffed Peppers

These little peppers look sophisticated, but the entire family will love eating them up.

Day Four

Breakfast: Goat Cheese and Veggie Scramble

This is the perfect savory breakfast. With the onions, tomatoes, peppers, eggs, and cheese you have the perfect well-rounded meal.

Lunch: Curried Chicken Salad

The Greek yogurt and mayo adds creaminess to the sandwich that you won't get anywhere else.

Dinner: Jamaican Pork Tenderloin with Beans

This is a quick summertime meal that everybody will love. Serve alongside some pilaf or brown rice.

Day Five

Breakfast: Superfood Smoothie

This four ingredient smoothie is quick to whip up and won't run you late.

Lunch: Tomato and Spinach Pasta

This dish is perfect for lunch or dinner. Make a double portion so you can have some later in the week.

Dinner: Grilled Turkey Burgers

It should never be said that you can't have a tasty and healthy burger. Fix some sweet potato fries to complete this meal.

RECIPES

Sides & Extras

Salsa

Ingredients:

- Salt

- 1 tbsp olive oil

- ½ lime

- 1 minced garlic clove

- 1/3 c coriander, chopped

- 1 jalapeno, chopped

- 1 onion, chopped

- 2 tomatoes, chopped

Instructions:

Mix everything together. Add salt to your taste. Allow refrigerating for 30 minutes.

Oven-Roasted Tomatoes

Ingredients:

salt

1 tbsp oil

4 thyme sprigs

1-pint Cherry tomatoes halved

Instructions:

The oven should be at 320. Place the tomatoes on a prepared baking sheet.
Top with salt and thyme and drizzle with oil. Cook for 45 minutes.

Zucchini Chips

Ingredients:

- salt

- 1 tbsp olive oil

- 4 zucchini, sliced

Instructions:

Place the zucchini slices on a prepared baking sheet. Top with oil and salt.

Cook for 30 minutes at 320 until they brown.

Breakfast

Basil and Tomato Frittata

Ingredients:

- ½ c Italian cheese, reduced-fat

- ¼ tsp pepper

- ¼ tsp salt

- 8 egg whites

- ¼ c basil, sliced

- 2 plum tomatoes

- 1 minced garlic clove

- 2 tsp EVOO

- ¼ c onion, chopped

Instructions:

Cook the onion in a hot skillet until it has become tender. Mix the garlic until fragrant. Stir in the tomato and cook until all the liquid is absorbed. Add in the basil.

Mix the pepper, salt, and eggs. Pour into the skillet over the veggies, and top with cheese. Slide the skillet into an oven that is set to broil. Cook until the eggs are set.

Pecan, Carrot, and Banana Muffin

Ingredients:

- ¼ c pecans, chopped

- 1 tsp vanilla

- ½ c banana, mashed

- ¾ c carrot, shredded

- 1/3 c yogurt, sugar-free

- 1 egg

- 1/3 c brown sugar

- ¼ c canola oil

- ½ tsp salt

- ¼ tsp baking soda

- 1 tsp cinnamon

- 1 tsp baking powder

- 1 c whole wheat flour

Instructions:

Mix the flour, baking powder, cinnamon, baking soda, and salt together.

Mix all the other ingredients, except for the nuts. Once combine, mix into the flour mixture. Gently fold in the pecans.

Pour into a prepared 6-cup muffin tin. In should bake for 22 minutes at 375.

Homemade Granola

Ingredients:

- ½ c brown sugar

- 1 ½ tsp salt

- ¼ c maple syrup

- ¾ c honey

- 1 c oil

- 2 tsp vanilla

- ½ c dried apricots

- ½ c sultans

- ½ c dried cranberries

- ½ c coconut flakes

- 1 c cashews

- 1 c walnuts

- ½ c flaked almonds

- 1 c pecans, chopped

- ½ c pepitas

- 1 c sunflower seeds

- 8 c rolled oats

Directions:

The oven should be at 325. Mix the nuts, coconut, and oats. In a pot mix the brown sugar, vanilla, sugar, oil, honey, maple syrup and allow to boil. Let it cook for five minutes until thick. Pour the sugar mixture over the nuts and quickly stir together.

Place the mixture on baking sheets lined with foil. Cook for 10 minutes. Remove and mix up the mixture. Bake for another 10 minutes. Once it's browned, mix in the dried fruits. Once cool, seal in a bowl or bag.

Goat Cheese and Veggie Scramble

Ingredients:

- ¼ c goat cheese

- ¼ tsp pepper

- ¼ tsp salt

- 1 c egg substitute

- ½ c tomato, chopped

- 2 tsp olive oil

- ¼ c onion, chopped

- ¼ c bell pepper, chopped

Instructions:

Cook the pepper and onion until soft. Mix in the tomato and cook until liquid is absorbed. Turn down the heat and add the egg substitute, pepper, and salt. Scramble the egg until cooked through. Top with goat cheese.

Superfood Smoothie

Instructions:

- 1 banana

- 2 c spinach

- 1 c blueberries, frozen

- 1 c almond milk

Instructions:

Place everything in your blender and mix until smooth.

Lunch

Carrot and Butternut Squash Soup

- ¼ cup half-and-half, fat-free

- ¼ tsp nutmeg

- ¼ tsp pepper

- 2 14 ½ -oz can chicken broth, reduced-sodium

- ¾ cup leeks, sliced

- 2 cup carrots, sliced

- 3 cup butternut squash, diced

- 1 tbsp butter

Instructions:

Melt the butter in a large pot. Place the leek, carrot, and squash in the hot

pot. Put on the lid, and allow to cook for about eight minutes. Pour in the

broth. Allow everything to come to boil. Turn down the heat to a simmer.

Place the lid on the pot and let cook for 25 minutes. The veggies should be

tender. With an immersion blender, mix the soup to the consistency that you

like. Season with the nutmeg and the pepper. Bring everything back to a boil

and stir in the half-and-half.

Lemony Hummus

Ingredients:

- ¼ c water

- 1 tbsp EVOO

- ¼ tsp cumin

- ¼ tsp pepper

- ½ tsp salt

- 1 clove garlic, chopped

- 1 ½ tbsp tahini

- ¼ c lemon juice

- 15-oz chickpeas, drained

Directions:

Add everything except for the water and oil in a food processor. Mix until combine. Add the oil and water and continue mixing until smooth. Add extra water if you need to.

Quinoa Tabbouleh

Ingredients:

- 2 scallions, sliced
- ½ c mint, chopped
- 2/3 c parsley
- 1-pint Cherry tomatoes
- 1 large cucumber
- pepper
- ½ c EVOO
- 1 minced garlic clove
- 2 tbsp lemon juice
- ½ tsp salt
- 1 c quinoa, rinsed

Instructions:

Cook the quinoa in salted water. As the quinoa cooks, mix the garlic and lemon juice. Slowly whisk in the EVOO, and then sprinkle with pepper and salt to your taste.

Allow the quinoa to cool completely. Toss with the dressing and then mix in the remaining ingredients. Add extra pepper and salt if needed.

Curried Chicken Salad

Ingredients:

- 4 whole wheat pita rounds

- 2 c mixed greens

- 1 c green grapes

- ¼ tsp pepper

- ¼ tsp salt

- 1 tsp curry powder

- 3 tbsp mayo, reduced-fat

- ½ c Greek yogurt, nonfat

- ¼ c slivered almonds

- 1 ¼-lb chicken, shredded

Instructions:

Mix all of the ingredients except for the greens and pitas. Divide the chicken

mixture into each pita. Top each with some greens.

Tomato and Spinach Pasta

Instructions:

- 3 tbsp parmesan, grated

- 1 tbsp balsamic vinegar

- ¼ tsp pepper

- 2 minced garlic cloves

- 1 c grape tomatoes

- 8 c spinach

- 2 tbsp olive oil

- 8-oz whole-wheat spaghetti

Instructions:

Cook the spaghetti the way the package says to, but without the salt. Drain.

As the pasta cooks, sauté the spinach until it wilts. Stir in the tomatoes and cook for about three minutes. Mix in the garlic.

Toss the pasta with the veggies and all the other ingredients.

Dinner

Grilled Shrimp Skewers

Ingredients:

- 9 skewers, soaked

- 1 lb cleaned shrimp

- 2 scallions, minced

- ¼ tsp pepper

- ½ tsp salt

- ¼ tsp red pepper flakes

- 1 medium lemon, zest, and juice

- 2 minced garlic cloves

- 1 ½ tbsp olive oil

Instructions:

Prepare your grill.

Mix the scallions, pepper, salt, pepper flakes, lemon juice and zest, garlic, and oil. Place the shrimp in the mixture and coat. Allow it to marinate in the refrigerate for 30 minutes.

Place the shrimp evenly among the skewers. Get rid on any remaining marinade.

Grill them shrimp until pink and firm, around two to three minutes.

Chicken Tortilla Soup

Ingredients:

- 1 c tortilla chips

- 2 minced garlic cloves

- 1 c chicken broth, reduced-sodium

- 2 c stir-fry veggies

- 2 c chicken, shredded

- 2 ½ c water

- 1 14 ½-oz can stewed tomatoes, Mexican-style

Directions:

In a crock pot, mix the garlic, broth, veggies, chicken, water, and

tomatoes. Cook for six and a half hours on low.

Top with chips.

Rice and Beef Stuffed Peppers

Ingredients:

- 1 tbsp parsley, divided

- ½ tsp pepper

- 2 tsp salt

- 4 minced garlic cloves

- ½ c tomato sauce

- ¼ c parsley

- ½ c Parmigiano-Reggiano, shredded

- 1 ½ c rice, cooked

- 1 ½ lb ground beef

- ¼ tsp red pepper flakes

- 1 c beef broth

- ½ onion, sliced

- 2 ½ c tomato sauce

- 6 bell peppers

Instructions:

The oven should be at 375. Cut the tops off the peppers and clean out the insides. Poke a few small holes in the bottom of each.

Place 2 ½ cups tomato sauce in a casserole dish. Place in the pepper flakes, broth, and onion. Set the peppers upright in the mixture.

Mix the pepper, salt, garlic, 2 tbsp tomato sauce, ¼ c parsley, cheese, rice, and beef. Divide the mixture between the peppers. Add a tablespoon of tomato sauce on top of each and lay the pepper tops back on. Top dish with parchment paper and then tin foil. Place the dish on a baking sheet.

Cook for an hour. They should be starting to feel soft. Take off the foil and parchment and cook for an addition 25 minutes.

Jamaican Pork Tenderloin

Ingredients:

- ½ tsp pepper
- ¼ tsp salt
- 1 tbsp lemon juice
- 1 tsp lemon zest
- 1 tbsp EVOO
- 1 lb green beans
- 3 c water
- 2 tbsp Creole mustard
- ¼ c grape jelly
- 2 tsp Jerk seasoning
- ¼ c orange juice, divided
- ¾ lb pork tenderloin

Instructions:

Mix the pepper, salt, lemon juice and zest, EVOO and water. Bring everything to a boil and add in the beans. As the beans cook, mix the mustard, jelly, jerk seasoning, and half the orange juice. Cover the tenderloin. The oven should be set and 350. Place the tenderloin in a casserole dish and pour in the rest of the orange juice. Bake for 45 minutes.

Grilled Turkey Burgers

Ingredients:

- 4 whole-wheat buns

- ½ tsp curry

- ¼ c Dijon

- 12-oz ground turkey

- 1/8 tsp pepper

- ¼ tsp garlic salt

- ¼ tsp Italian seasoning

- 2 tbsp milk, fat-free

- 2 tbsp bread crumbs

- ¼ c green onions, sliced

- ½ c carrot, shredded

Instructions:

Mix the ground turkey with the seasonings, bread crumbs, and veggies.

Form the meat mixture into four patties.

Prepare your grill, and cook the patties until done. Mix the mustard and curry powder and spread onto the buns. Add the burgers to the buns. Top with tomato and lettuce if desired.

Dessert

Blueberries and Yogurt

Ingredients:

1/3 c Greek yogurt

10 blueberries

Instructions:

Top the yogurt with the blueberries and enjoy.

Raspberry Sorbet

Ingredients:

- lemon juice
- 1 c raspberries

Instructions:

Place the ingredients in a food processor and mix until smooth. Place in an airtight container and freeze.

PART II

Chapter 1: Diabetes and A Realistic Diet Plan

Suffering from the symptoms of diabetes doesn't have to be as complicated as some believe it is if you provide a daily healthier diet outlook on the foods you consume. You can help 'ward-off' the complications with a healthy eating plan which can control your blood sugar, while at the same time help lower your risks of heart disease and cancer. These are some of the ways a healthy diet can improve your life:

Improves Your Overall Health

The amount of inflammation in your body can be reduced with a healthy diet—as well as decreasing the triglycerides, bad cholesterol {LDL}; it also increases the good cholesterol {HDL}.

Another diabetic complication, metabolic syndrome, is remedied with healthy carbohydrate sources in foods such as olive oil, nuts, and lean protein choices. The condition is presented with many conditions including elevated, blood sugar, blood pressure, and cholesterol which are all stressors that work as a team to cause issues including diabetes, strokes, and heart disease.

The Link between Strokes and Diabetes

For individuals who have diabetes; you are also at a greater risk for strokes and heart disease.Research provided by the American Heart Association indicates that at least 65% of the patients who have diabetes, also die from strokes and heart disease.

This factor may be that the patients did not consume a healthy diet and often become sedentary and obese from the lack of energy and activity.

Components of a Health Diabetic Diet Plan

These are the food groups you should be most concerned with as a person with diabetes. As you will see, throughout this list and the provided recipes; you don't have to deprive yourself of the foods you enjoy. You just need to learn how to prepare and group them together. You will need to make some adjustments, but it is worth it.

These are the food groups you should consider as part of your diabetic plan:

1. *Whole Grains*: Oats, bulgar, brown rice, barley whole grain cereals, and bread, as well as whole wheat pasta.

2. *Vegetables and fruits*

3. *Low-fat or fat-free dairy products*: Milk, cheese, and yogurt

4. *Unsaturated fats*: Nuts in moderate amounts and vegetable oils {Limit unhealthy trans fats and saturated fats, salt, and sugar}

5. *Lean Proteins:* Fish, skinless poultry, lean cuts of beef, and beans

These are the elements that the healthier diet will play in lowering your risk of diabetes complications:

Fresh Produce: Vegetables and fruits will provide many minerals and vitamins as well as being an excellent source of fiber. Blood glucose control and weight management are better maintained with the lower calorie content.

Fiber: Your blood sugar management, heart health, and digestion depend on fiber. The fiber can raise the sugar/glucose levels, lower the cholesterol levels, and satisfy your hunger for longer times.

Low-fat Dairy: You can acquire excellent sources of potassium which is essential to prevent the risk of osteoporosis, a thinning/weakness of the bones making them more prone to fractures. It is documented that individuals with diabetes are more likely to be at risk for these issues which make a healthier diet a reasonable step to take in the ways of prevention.

Lean Proteins: Your body will be more sensitive to producing its insulin when you
provide the leaner choices protein. As a result, you can lower the risk of heart disease and excessive weight gain.

The Myths

Today's society is in such a churn that is sometimes difficult to realize you need a special diet until it's too late. The onset of diabetes is on the rise, but so many cases can be reversed, and some are preventable. First, and foremost, you will soon understand the essence of a good recipe guide. However, you need to dispel some of the myths involved with the disease and a diet plan. These are some of the myths about dieting and diabetes:

- *Myth #1:* Avoid sugar at all costs.

- *Fact #1:* The primary element you need to consider is to limit and properly plan the hidden sugars. Make the dessert a part of the healthy meal plan. You will notice there are several yummy choices in the recipe section.

- *Myth #2:* You will need special diabetic meals.

- *Fact #2:* Everyone eats the same foods if you are following a healthy diet—diabetic—or not. Purchasing specific foods for 'diabetics only' is essentially a waste of money {generally speaking}. After all, do you know what is packaged in the box? Many times the food has the forbidden 'hidden sugars.' Do you have time to shop and look at every ingredient on the label? Probably not.

- *Myth #3:* You have to cut way back on your carbohydrate intake.

- *Fact #3:* You need to consider the kind of carbs you are consuming; remembering the serving size is the key element. Eliminate the starchy carbs and focus on the whole grain carbs since they are digested slower and are high in fiber. It will help keep the blood sugar levels on an even kilter.

Chapter 2: Wake – Up With a Healthy Start

These are just a few of the ways you can begin your day. Some of the recipe ideas can be prepared in advance. Enjoy!

Banana & Grapefruit

This delicious bowl of 'chilly' bites will surprise you!

Ingredients

1 Tablespoon freshly chopped mint

1 cup sliced banana {approximately one}

1 {24-ounces} Jar of red grapefruit sections

1 Tablespoon honey

1. Drain and save ¼ cup of the grapefruit juice.
2. Combine the entire batch of ingredients in a medium serving dish.
3. Toss and serve or cover and chill.

Be ready in the morning, and prepare this the night before. You can even make it easily transportable.

Yields: Three {1-cup servings}

Oat Pancakes

Ingredients

1 Cup oat flour

¼ Cup artificial sweetener

1 teaspoon baking powder

¼ Cup rolled oats

1 Tablespoon each:

- Ginger

- Cinnamon

1 egg/egg substitute equivalent

½ cup low-fat milk

1 teaspoon vanilla extract

Directions

1. Prepare the griddle to 275°F.

2. Combine all of the dry ingredients and then add the wet components—mixing thoroughly.

3. Cook them as a regular pancake; waiting for the bubbles to mount up before you flip them. Always check the bottom to see if it is browned to your liking before you turn the pancake over.

Notes: You can also add some blueberries which you can sprinkle on top of the batter when it is poured onto the griddle, so you don't pop them open in the mixing process. Try adding some fruit or nuts to the mixture.

Rosemary Omelet and Veggies

Ingredients

2 Tbsp. Water

¾ cup refrigerated egg product {Ex. Egg Beaters}

¼ cup sharp cheddar cheese {shredded & reduced-fat} 1

{12-ounce} Frozen Red Potatoes {Cook-in-the-Bag}

    With added Green beans with rosemary butter sauce

Fresh chives

1. Prepare the veggies according to the package instructions.

2. Use some cooking spray and lightly coat a skillet—preheating it to the medium-high setting.

3. Whisk the water and egg product in a small container and pour into the prepared skillet. Let it cook undisturbed—allowing it to set. Run the spatula around the edges so that the uncooked egg will flow downward to the pan for about 30 to 60 seconds. When the mixture is set—turn off the heat.

4. Place the veggies in a nine-inch microwavable pie plate, and add the omelet to the top while folding {tucking} in the edges around the plate.

5. Sprinkle with the cheese and microwave on high {100%} power until the cheese melts, usually about thirty seconds.

Note: Green Giant Steamers brand is an excellent choice.

Yields: Three servings {One serving = 1/3 of an omelet and ½ cup of veggies}

Grams of Carbs per Serving: 18

Yogurt Pudding

Ingredients

¼ Cup Crushed Pineapple {Can – juice pack}

1 {6-ounces} Carton vanilla low-fat yogurt

½ Cup fat-free milk

½ Cup regular rolled oats

½ teaspoon vanilla

1 tablespoon flax seed meal/chia seeds

Optional:

1/8 teaspoon toasted sliced almonds

Directions

1. Combine the pineapple, yogurt, vanilla, chia seeds, cinnamon, milk, and oats in a medium dish. Add them to a container and secure the lid.

2. Chill in the fridge for two days or at least for eight hours.

3. Stir completely, and add the almonds, if desired, as well as the apple.

Yields: Two Servings {3/4 Cup each}

Grams of Carbs per Serving: 38

Baked Apple

Ingredients

1 Cup Fresca

1 Tablespoon cornstarch

¼ teaspoon cinnamon

1 ½ teaspoon sweetener substitute

¼ teaspoon salt

Apples

Butter for the tops of apples

1. Cut the apples in half and remove the seeds.

2. Preheat the oven to 375°F.

3. Combine the cinnamon, salt, and cornstarch with 1 Tablespoon of Fresca.

4. Stir as you gradually add the remainder of the Fresca until it is clear and smooth.

5. Arrange the halved apples in a baking dish and empty the mixture over them while dotting each one with the butter.

6. Bake for 45 minutes to about an hour.

Apple Jelly

You will love the fact you know what is in your jelly when you make it from scratch. This one is a winner!

Ingredients

2 Packages unflavored gelatin

4 Tablespoons artificial sweetener

1-quart apple juice

2 Tablespoons lemon juice

Directions

1. Mix all of the components on the list in a saucepan and blend well.

2. All you need to do is boil the jelly for about five minutes. Let it cool.

3. Pour into the containers and store in the fridge.

Chapter 3: Mid-Day Recipes

Along about mid-day, you are probably in need of a healthy 'pick-me-up.' These are some of the ways you can get going for the rest of the day.

Barbecue Ranch Wraps

Ingredients

1 -Tablespoon salad dressing/light mayonnaise

2 - Tablespoons Ranch salad dressing {reduced-fat}

2 Cups packaged shredded broccoli/slaw mix type

4 {8-inches} Whole grain flour tortillas

8 ounces cooked turkey or chicken breasts

2 Tablespoons Barbecue Sauce

Directions

1.   Combine the mayonnaise and ranch dressing in a medium mixing dish; blend in the broccoli.

2.   Cover the tortillas with a layer of the barbecue sauce.

3.   Top it off with the chicken and broccoli mixture.

Roll them up.

Yields: Four Servings

Diabetic & Heart-Healthy Stuffed Peppers

Ingredients

4 Tablespoons Corn oil

2 garlic cloves

2 sliced onions

4 diced tomatoes

1 diced zucchini

2 cups brown rice {cooked}

4 large seeded green peppers

½ cup grated cheddar cheese

2 cups tomato juice

1. Set the oven in advance to 375°F.

2. Prepare a large pan with the oil using medium heat.

3. Sauté the tomatoes, zucchini, onions, and garlic; until they are done. Add the rice and cheese to the pan.

4. Stuff the peppers with the veggie mixture and put the tops back on.

5. Empty the juice into the bottom of a casserole dish/pan and bake for 30 minutes.

Yields: Four Servings

Hummus and Avocado Salad Sandwiches

Ingredients

½ of an avocado {peeled and sliced}

1/3 Cup Mediterranean-flavor hummus

¼ teaspoon black pepper

1 Cup Arugula leaves

4 - whole wheat, split bagel bread or sandwich thins

½ Cup or {2-ounces} Gruyere cheese

1. Lightly grease a skillet with a small amount of cooking spray.

2. Heat the pan on the medium temperature setting or use the outdoor grill.

3. Spread some of the hummus on each of the bagel thins, and sprinkle with the pepper.

4. Begin the layer of the sandwich with the avocado slices, arugula, and shredded cheese. Place the tops on with the spread-side down, and put them on the skillet/grill.

5. Toast them for about two minutes with another object/skillet on top to keep the sandwich firm {like they use at the Waffle House}. Flip the sandwich and cook another two minutes.

Yields: Four Servings {One sandwich}

Grams of Carbs per Serving: 26

Beef and Bean Chili

Ingredients

1 Cup finely chopped onions

2 Pounds ground beef

2 medium carrots

1 can tomato paste

1 {28-ounces} Can of tomatoes – undrained and chopped

1 {16-ounces} Can kidney or pinto

beans Chili Seasoning

Mild grated cheese

1. Peel and grate the carrots.
2. Prepare the beef and onions in a skillet until done, and drain the grease.
3. Combine the remainder of the ingredients with the mixture— excluding the beans.
4. Let the ingredients blend in the skillet for approximately 45 minutes, and add the beans—cooking until they are warmed.

Serve in a bowl with a topping of cheese.

Enjoy with some crackers or homemade cornbread!

Yields: 2 ½ quarts

Chicken Salad with Orzo

Ingredients

1 Cup frozen/fresh corn kernels

2/3 Cup dried {3-ounces} orzo pasta

2 cups chopped/shredded cooked chicken breast

¼ Cup Freshly cut cilantro 1

Cup halved grape tomatoes

½ Cup {2-ounces reduced-fat} Feta cheese

1. Prepare the orzo—adding the corn the last minute of the cooking time. It will cool quickly by rinsing with cold water; Drain.
2. Mix the chicken orzo mixture, cilantro, and tomatoes in a large serving bowl. Give them a sprinkle of crumbled cheese.
3. Place them in the refrigerator for a minimum of two hours— preferably 24-hours.
4. Drizzle with your favorite dressing.

Yields: Four Servings {1/4 Cup dressing and 1 Cup salad}

Grams of Carbs per Serving: 30

Salmon Tacos

Ingredients

14 to 16 ounces cooked salmon

1 Tbsp. Lime juice

8 {6-inch} warmed tortillas

½ C. thinly sliced red sweet pepper

1 C. shredded cabbage with carrots

1 *Sour Cream Drizzle* recipe {below}

Lime Wedges {*Optional*}

1. Gently toss the cooked salmon with the juice of the lime until saturated.
2. Add the sweet peppers, cabbage, and salmon mixture to floured tortilla.
3. Garnish each one of the tortillas with a drizzle of the sour cream or sprinkle with some cilantro, and serve with a lime wedge or two.

Note: You can substitute coleslaw mix in this recipe for the cabbage mixture.

Yields: Four Servings {2 Tacos}

Grams of Carbs per Serving: 27

For the Sour Cream Drizzle:

1 Tbsp. Lime juice

1 Tbsp. Fresh cilantro

1/3 C. light sour cream

1/8 tsp. each:

- Salt

- chili powder

Thoroughly mix all of the listed ingredients in a mixing bowl.

Chapter 4: Dinner Time

Here are some ideas for dinner time which cover several choices:

Beef

Beef Burgundy

Ingredients

2 Pounds Top round steak

½ Cup dry - red wine

1 Tbsp. flour

1 Pouch onion soup mix {dry}

1 {3-ounces} Can mushrooms

1 ¾ - Cups water

1. Heat the oven to 350°F.

2. Slice the steak into one-inch cubes.

3. Prepare a skillet with a small amount of vegetable spray. Add the beef
    and cook slowly.

4. Drain and place the meat into a 1 ½ quart casserole dish with a
    tight-fitting lid.

5. Combine and add the remainder of the ingredients—stirring well.

6. Cover the dish and bake for 15 additional minutes

You can serve over some noodles or rice. What a yummy delight!

Cabbage Rolls

Ingredients

3 ounces ground beef

1 large cabbage leaf

2 minced onions

1 teaspoon tomato sauce or diabetic ketchup

1 tablespoon minced green pepper

Directions

1. Heat the oven to 350°F.

2. Prepare the beef, and add the onions and green peppers for about the last five minutes.

3. Drain the ingredients and mix in the seasonings.

4. Put the components into the cabbage leaf and roll. Use a toothpick to close the leaf.

5. Bake for a short time until the cabbage leaf is cooked to the desired doneness.

Chipotle Meatloaf with Cilantro

Ingredients

1/2 {10-ounces} Package frozen-cooked brown rice – thawed—{approx. 1 ½

Cups}

2/3 Cup Chipotle salsa

¼ Cup frozen/refrigerated egg product {thawed}

2 Tablespoons ground flax seed meal

1 Lb. Ex.-lean ground beef

¾ Cup chopped fresh cilantro

¼ teaspoon salt

1. Set the oven temperature to 350°F.

2. Line a baking pan with foil and cooking spray.

3. Mix the egg product, 2/3 of the salsa, salt, cilantro, and rice; lastly, add the beef and mix well.

4. Make, and place the meat mixture into a loaf pan. Bake for 40 to 45 minutes or 160°F with a thermometer.

5. Remove the tasty meatloaf from the oven and spoon the remainder of the salsa onto the top. Let it rest for about ten minutes.

Yields: 4 {7-ounces) Servings

Grams of Carbs per Serving: 15

Chicken

Chicken Breasts & Orange Sauce

Ingredients

1 ½ Pounds Chicken breasts {no bones or skin}

½ teaspoon each:

- Paprika

- Tarragon

1 teaspoon salt

4 teaspoons unsaturated butter

1 Cup orange juice

1 sliced orange

1 Tablespoon grated orange rind

1. Flavor the chicken with the pepper and salt.

2. Arrange the chicken in a casserole container and brown with the butter.

3. Add the juice, tarragon, and rind. Bake in an uncovered dish for thirty minutes.

4. Take the meal from the oven, and put the pan with the liquid/juices back in the oven. Increase the heat to thicken the sauce.

5. Enjoy the flavorsome sauce over some steamed rice or just over the chicken. Garnish with an orange slice or two.

Baked Chicken and Rice

Ingredients

6 halves chicken breast {no skin}

1 Package onion soup mix {divided}

1 Cup cooked rice

1/8 teaspoon pepper

1 Can {10- ¾ ounces} Cream of mushroom soup

1 ½ - Cups water

Directions

1. Heat the oven to 325°F.

2. Arrange the rice on the bottom of a rectangular baking dish/pan; a 9 x 12 would work nicely.

3. Use ¼ of the soup mix, and drizzle it over the rice; add the chicken, and sprinkle the remainder of the mix along with the pepper, water, and can of soup. Stir well.

4. Pour the soup over the breasts of chicken.

5. Cover the dish and bake for approximately two hours.

Chicken Cacciatora

Ingredients

3 {1/2-Pounds} skinless chicken breast

1 garlic clove

1 tsp. oregano

2 Tbsp. Olive oil

1 {16-ounces} Can stewed tomatoes

1 ½ C. sliced mushrooms

Optional:

- Parsley

- Pepper

- Salt

1. Pour the oil in a skillet and brown the chicken with the garlic. Give it a sprinkle of pepper, salt, and oregano before you flip it over to the other side. Discard the garlic.

2. Toss in the mushrooms until lightly browned, and pour in the tomatoes.

3. Place a top on the pan and cook for about thirty minutes, and uncover.

4. Continue to cook until the sauce is the desired consistency.

5. Top it off with some parsley.

Chicken Teriyaki

Ingredients

1 Skinned broiler-fryer

1 teaspoon each:

- Dry mustard

- Ginger

- Garlic salt

½ Cup Soy Sauce

2 Tablespoons each:

- Brown sugar substitute

- Lemon juice

- Water

1. Mix together all of the ingredients—omit the chicken—in a small pan and boil.

2. Empty the contents over the chicken into a container and marinate it in the fridge for about two or more hours {a plastic baggie is excellent}.

3. You can either bake in the oven or use the grill. Use the tasty sauce for basting during the cooking process.

4. *Note: Cook in the Microwave*: 10 minutes; turn and cook ten more.

Oven-Fried Chicken

Ingredients

1 Cut-up Fryer

¼ cup each:

- Buttermilk

- Wheat germ

- Potato flakes

½ teaspoon each:

- Garlic salt

- Salt

- Paprika

Pinch of Pepper

1. Set the oven in advance to 350°F. Lightly grease a baking dish with some cooking spray.

2. Flavor the fryer with some pepper and salt, and let it rest to blend about half an hour or more.

3. Dip it into the buttermilk. Then into this mixture—potato flakes, wheat germ, paprika, and garlic salt.

4. Arrange the chicken in the dish and bake for approximately 35 minutes.

Fish

Baby Shrimp and Mustard Tarragon Dip

Ingredients

1 C. baby shrimp

2 tsp. dried tarragon

1 tsp. lemon juice

1 C. mayonnaise

1 ½ - tsp. white wine vinegar

2 Tbsp. Dijon mustard

½ cup sour cream

1. Combine the tarragon, mustard, vinegar, and lemon juice.

2. Blend the mayonnaise into the mixture and add the shrimp—followed by the sour cream.

3. Blend the ingredients well—cover—and chill.

Yields: Ten Servings

Grams of Carbs per Serving: 1

Tuna Casserole

Ingredients

1 Can Chow Mein noodles

1 Can diabetic tuna fish

1 Can cream of mushroom soup

1 Cup water

Pepper and salt

Topping: Cubes of butter

Directions

1. Set the temperature in the oven to 350°F.

2. Mix all of the components.

3. Bake for one hour.

Have some fresh rolls to complement this tasty dish.

Pork

Saucy Thai

Ingredients

1 {14-ounces} Package Frozen sweet pepper stir-fry vegetables

1 Pound Boneless pork loin

½ C. Unsweetened coconut milk {reduced-fat}

3 tsp. olive oil {divided}

1 1/3 C. brown rice {cooked}

1 Tbsp. of Each:

- All-purpose flour

- Thai-style seasoning blend

1. Thaw and drain the veggies. Trim away any fat and cut the pork into bite-size pieces; set aside.

2. Whisk the coconut milk, Thai seasoning, and flour together and set to the side.

3. In the meantime, pour one teaspoon of the oil in a pan using the medium heat setting. Toss in the veggies and cook—covered for three to five minutes until crispy but tender. When it is done; place them in a separate container.

4. Pour the remainder of the oil in the skillet and add the pork. Cook over the med-high setting for three to five minutes. Put the vegetables back into the skillet.

5. Blend in the coconut milk mixture and continue cooking until the sauce has thickened, for one to two minutes; stir frequently.

6. Serve over a nice plate of hot cooked rice.

Yields: Four servings {1/3 cup of rice plus ¾ cup pork mixture}

Grams of Carbs per Serving: 23

Pork Chops and Apples

Ingredients

1 medium chopped onion

4 lean-cut pork chops

¼ teaspoon pepper

1 teaspoon pepper

1 ¼ Cups Water

½ teaspoon cinnamon

3 Medium cooking apples

Directions

1. Peel and slice the apples.

2. Brown the chops and onions in a skillet.

3. Mix water, pepper along with the bouillon in a mixing dish. Add this to the skillet. Cover and let it boil.

4. Lower the heat and continue cooking for approximately twenty minutes.

5. Remove/skim away the fat and add the apples and cinnamon.

6. Cover the meat and simmer about fifteen more minutes and serve piping hot.

Pork Chops and Gravy

Ingredients

1 Can cream of mushroom soup

2 Tablespoons flour

4 small pork chops

Optional:

- Parsley

- Pepper

1. Set the oven temperature in advance to 350°F.

2. Flavor the chops lightly with the pepper and coat them with the flour.

3. Use some cooking spray to coat a baking dish, and add the pork.

4. Empty the soup over the pork chops along with the water. {You can blend them together beforehand if you wish to make it easier.}

5. Sprinkle with the parsley {if desired}.

6. Secure the lid or use some heavy-duty foil, and bake for about 1- to 1 ½ hours.

Enjoy with some rice or potatoes.

Chapter 5: Tasty Snacks

These are several items you can enjoy when you cannot resist the urge for something sweet!

Applesauce Cake

Ingredients

1 Cup unsweetened applesauce

2 Cups Each:

- Water

- Raisins

2 T. liquid sweetener

¾ Cup oil

2 eggs

2 Cups flour

¼ tsp. nutmeg

1 tsp. baking soda

1 tsp. vanilla

Directions

1. Preheat the oven to 350°F. Prepare a loaf pan with some cooking spray.

2. Add the raisins to the water and cook until the water is absorbed.

3. Put the eggs, applesauce, sweetener, and oil once the raisins are cool. Blend well.

4. Sift in the soda, nutmeg, and flour. Add the vanilla and combine.

5. Empty the batter into the baking pan and bake for approximately one hour.

Banana Bread

Ingredients

4 tsp. baking powder

½ Cup Splenda®

1 tsp. each:

- salt

- baking powder

2 ½ Cups all-purpose {un-sifted}

1/3 Cup polyunsaturated butter

1 Cup mashed ripe bananas

2 {stiffly beaten} egg whites

½ Cup skim milk

Directions

1. Prepare the oven setting to 350°F. Lightly grease a loaf pan.

2. Mix the flour, Splenda, baking powder, and salt—blending well.

3. Add the milk, beaten eggs, butter, and bananas.

4. Mix using an electric mixer for one minute at the low-speed setting.

5. Pour the prepared batter into the loaf pan.

6. Place in the preheated oven for 55 to 60 minutes.

Rice Pudding

Ingredients

1 Package Instant sugar-free pudding

1 Cup Cooked Rice

2 Cups Water

1 cup of milk

Optional:

- Cinnamon

- Raisins

Directions

1. Prepare the pudding by adding the above ingredients together.

2. Add the mixture to the rice, and enjoy. {Guilt-Free}

Beverages

Chilly Berry

You will love this tasty delight and not feel guilty!

Ingredients

1 {12-ounces} Can Strawberry/Cherry carbonated beverage {sugar-free}

1/3 Cup Unsweetened pineapple juice

½ Cup Strawberry ice cream

Directions

1. Use a pretty, tall glass, add the chilled ingredients, and enjoy!

Garnish with a mint leaf and a sliced berry.

Orange & Cream Punch

Ingredients

1 2/3 Cups diabetic sweetener {Splenda}

1 Package unsweetened orange drink {Kool-Aid®}

1/3 teaspoon vanilla {to taste}

Directions

1. Combine the Splenda and drink mix and add to a two-quart pitcher.

2. Add the water to the fill line and stir well. Add the vanilla, and stir again.

3. Place a lid on the pitcher and let it chill in the fridge for two to four hours. You want it super cold.

4. Add a lemon slice and some ice; enjoy!

Sparkling Fruit Drink

Ingredients

1 Quart diet ginger ale

Ice

8 Ounces Each Unsweetened:

- Orange juice

- Grape juice

- Apple juice

Directions

1. Mix the ingredients together and add the ice cubes.

Yields: Seven Servings {Nine-ounces each}

Index for the Recipes

Chapter 2: Wake – Up With a Healthy Start

Chapter 3: Mid-Day Recipes

Chapter 4: Dinner Time

Beef

- Beef Burgundy

- Cabbage Rolls

- Chipotle Meatloaf with Cilantro

Chicken

- Chicken Breasts & Orange Sauce

- Baked Chicken and Rice

- Chicken Cacciatora

- Chicken Teriyaki

- Oven-Fried Chicken

Fish

- Baby Shrimp and Mustard Tarragon Dip

- Tuna Casserole

Pork

- Saucy Thai

- Pork Chops and Apples

- Pork Chops and Gravy

Chapter 5: Tasty Snacks

- Applesauce Cake

- Banana Bread

- Rice Pudding

Beverages

- Chilly Berry

- Orange & Cream Punch

- Sparkling Fruit Punch

PART III

Chapter 1: What Is Fasting?

Introduction to Fasting

Latest Research and Studies about Fasting

In a research published by the Springer Journal, it was found that fasting helps fight against obesity. The study, led by Kyoung Han Kim and Yun Hye Kim, was aimed at tracking the effects of fasting on fat cells. They put a group of mice into a four-month period of intermittent fasts, where the mice were fed for two days, followed by a day of fasting. In the end, the group of fasting mice was found to weigh less than the non-fasting mice, even though all of them had consumed exact quantities of food. The group of fasting mice had registered a drop in the fat buildup around fat cells. The explanation was that the fat had been converted into energy when glucose was insufficient. (www.sciencedaily.com/releases/2017/10/171017110041.htm)

In November 2017, Harvard researchers established that fasting can induce a long life, as well as minimize aging effects. It was found that fasting revitalizes mitochondria. Mitochondria are the organelles that act as body power plants. In this replenished state, mitochondria optimize physiological functions, in effect slowing down the aging process. Fasting also promotes low blood glucose levels, which improves skin clarity and boosts the immune system. (https://newatlas.com/fasting-increase-lifespan-mitochondria-harvard/52058/)

Sebastian Brandhorst, a researcher based at the University of Southern California, found out that fasting has a positive impact on brain health. Fasting induces low blood sugar levels, causing the liver to produce ketone bodies that pass on to the brain in place of sugars. Ketone bodies are much more stable and efficient energy sources than glucose. Researchers from the same university have posited that fasting minimizes chances of coming down with diabetes and other degenerative diseases. Moreover, they discovered that fasting induces low production of the IGF-1 hormone, which is a catalyst in aging and spread of disease. (https://www.cnbc.com/2017/10/20/science-diet-fasting-may-be-more-important-than-just-eating-less.html)

Biological Effects of Fasting
- **Cleanses the body**

Our bodies harbor an endless count of toxins, and these toxins announce their presence through symptoms like low energy, infections, allergies, terrible moods, bloating, confusion, and so on.

Eliminating toxins from your body will do you a world of good in the sense that your body will upgrade and start functioning optimally. There are many ways to cleanse your body: hydrotherapy, meditation, organic diets, herbs, yoga, etc.

But one of the most effective ways of cleansing your body is through fasting. When you go on a fast, you allow the body to channel the energy that would have been used for digestion into flushing out toxins.

- **Improves heart health**

Studies show that people who undertake regular fasts are less likely to contract coronary infections. Fasting fights against obesity, and obesity is a recipe for heart disease. It purifies the blood too, in that sense augmenting the flow of blood around the body.

- **Improves the immune system**

Fasting rids the body of toxins and radicals, thus boosting the body's immune system and minimizes the chances of coming down with degenerative diseases like cancer. Fasting reduces inflammation as well.

- **Improves bowel movement**

One of the problems of consuming food on the regular is that the food sort of clogs up your stomach, causing indigestion. You might go for days without visiting the bathroom to perform number two. But when you fast, your body resources won't be bogged down by loads of undigested foods, and so your bowel movement will be seamless. Also, fasting promotes healthy gut bacteria.

- **Induces alertness**

When your stomach is full because of combined undigested foods (i.e., "garbage"), you are more likely to experience brain-fog. You won't have any concentration on the tasks at hand. You will just sit around and laze the hours away, belching and spitting. But when you fast, your mind will be clear so it will be easy to cultivate focus.

Treating Fasting as a Lifestyle Choice

When you perform a simple Google search for the word "fasting," millions of results come up. Fasting is slowly becoming a mainstream subject. This is mostly because of the research-backed evidence that has been published by many reputable publications listing down the various benefits of fasting such as improved brain health, increased production of the human growth hormone, a stronger immune system, heart health, and weight loss—thus its appeal to health-conscious people as a catalyst for their health goals.

Taking up fasting as a lifestyle choice will see you go without food for anywhere from a couple of hours to days. But before you get into it, you'd do yourself a world of good to first obtain clearance from a physician, certifying that your body is ready, because not everyone is made for it. For instance, the symptoms of illnesses such as cancer may worsen after a long stretch of food deprivation. So people with degenerative diseases such as cancer should consider getting professional help or staying away altogether. Pregnant women, malnourished people, and children are advised to stay clear too.

The first thing you must do is to establish your fasting routine. For instance, you may choose to skip breakfast, making lunch your first meal of the day. Go at it with consistency. Also, you may decide to space your meals over some hours; so that when the set hours elapse, you reach your eating window, and then go back to fasting. The real challenge is staying committed. You will find that it will be difficult to break the cycle of eating that your body had been accustomed to, but when you persevere; your body will, of course, adjust to your new habit. If you decide to go for days without food, the results will be far pronounced, but please remember to hydrate your body constantly to flush out toxins.

Summary

Fasting is the willing abstinence from food over a period of time with the goal of improving your life. Conventionally, fasting has been tied to religious practices, but a new school of thought has emerged to proclaim the health benefits of fasting—particularly, weight loss. When you go into a fast, you create a caloric deficit, which triggers the body to convert its fat stores into energy. Numerous studies by mainstream health organizations have been done on fasting, and researchers have established that fasting has a host of advantages like improved motor skills, cognition, and moods. Some of the biological effects of fasting include improved bowel movement, immune system, and heart health. If you are starting out with fasting, you must create a routine and abide by it. Not everyone is fit to practice fasting. Some of the people advised to stay away from the practice include extremely sick people, pregnant women, the malnourished, and children. If you undertake a prolonged fast, you should hydrate your body constantly.

Chapter 2: Obesity and the Standard American Diet

The Obesity Epidemic

We are killing ourselves with nothing more than a spoon and a fork. In 2017, obesity claimed more lives than car accidents, terrorism, and Alzheimer's combined. And the numbers are climbing at a jaw-dropping rate. Obesity has become a crisis that we cannot afford to ignore anymore.

You'd be mistaken to think that obesity is a crisis in first-world economies alone. Even developing nations are experiencing an upsurge of obese citizens. Here comes the big question: what is the **main** force behind this epidemic?

According to new research published in the New England Journal of Medicine, excessive caloric intake and lack of exercise are to blame.

Most American fast food chains have now become global. Fast foods, which are particularly calorie-laden, appeal to a lot of people across the world because of their low prices and taste. So, most people get hooked on the fast food diet and slowly begin the plunge into obesity.

The United States recognizes obesity as a health crisis and lawmakers have petitioned for tax increment on fast foods and sugary drinks, except that for a person who's addicted to fast foods, it would take a lot more than a price increase to discourage their food addiction. It would take a total lifestyle change.

Exercising alone won't help you; no matter how powerful your reps may be, or leg lifts or anything else you try in the gym, nothing can save you from a terrible diet.

And here's the complete shocker; the rate of childhood obesity has surpassed adulthood obesity; a terrible, terrible situation considering that childhood obesity almost always leads to heart complications in adult life.

Why Are We So Fat?

- **Poor food choices**

The number one reason why we are so fat is our poor choice of food. We eat too much of the wrong food, and most of it is not expended, so it becomes stored up as fat.

- **Bad genetics**

It's true that some people are genetically predisposed to gain more weight. Their genetics have wired them to convey abnormal hunger signals, so their bodies pressure them into consuming much more food.

- **Lack of strenuous activities**

Our modern-day lives involve only light physical tasks. Contrast that with the era of the dawn of humanity. Back then people would use up a lot of energy to perform physical activities and survive in unforgiving habitats.

Most of the food they consumed would be actually utilized. But today, thanks to our technological advancement, we have been spared from taking part in laborious activities. This makes it hard to use up the energy from food, and the body opts to store it as fat.

- **Psychological issues**

Some of us react to bad moods by indulging in food—in particular, high-calorie fast foods—because the taste of fast foods appeals to our unstable emotions. When we fall in the habit of rewarding our bad moods or depression with binge eating, we unsuspectingly fall into the trap of food addiction, to the point of getting depressed when we fail to binge eat, kicking off our journey into obesity.

- **The endocrine system**

The thyroid's hormones play a critical role in the metabolic rate of a person. Ideally, a strong endocrine system means a high metabolic rate. And so, individuals who have a weakened endocrine system are much more likely to develop obesity.

The Problem with Calories

Calories are the basic units for quantifying the energy in the food we consume. A healthy man needs a daily dose of around 2500 calories to function optimally, and a woman needs 2000 calories.

This caloric target should be met through the consumption of various foods containing minerals, vitamins, antioxidants, fiber, and other important elements, and this is not hard at all to achieve if you adhere to the old-fashioned "traditional diet."

But the challenge is that nowadays, we have many foods with a high caloric count, and yet they hardly fill us up! For instance, fries, milkshake, and a burger make up nearly 2000 calories! You can see how easy it'd be to surpass the caloric limit by indulging in fast food.

When we consume more calories than we burn, our bodies store up the excess calories as fat, and as this process repeats itself over time, the fat has a compounding effect that leads to weight gain.

The only way to make your weight stable is through balancing out the energy you consume with the energy you expend. But for someone who suffers from obesity, if they'd like to have a normal weight, they must create a caloric deficit, and fasting is the surefire practice of creating such a deficit.

Besides checking your caloric intake, you might also consider improving your endocrine system and the efficiency of both your kidney and liver, because they have a direct impact on how the body burns calories. When you buy food products, always find out their caloric count to assess how well they'll fit within your daily caloric needs.

The American Diet

In a 2016 lifestyle survey, most Americans admitted that it is not easy to keep their diet clean and healthy. This isn't surprising, especially when you consider the fact that the average American consumes more than 20 pounds of sweeteners each year. The over-emphasis of sugar and fat in the American diet is the leading cause of obesity in Americans. Illnesses triggered by obesity long started marching into our homes. What we have now is a crisis. But let's find out the exact types of foods that Americans like to feast on (we are big on consuming, it's no secret).

As a melting point of cultures drawn from various parts of the world, it's kind of difficult to say exactly what the all-American favorite foods are. But the United States Department of Agriculture might shine some light on this. It listed down desserts, bread, chicken, soda, and alcohol, as the top five sources of calories among Americans. As you can see, the sugar intake is impossibly high. Interestingly, the US Department of Agriculture also noted that Americans aren't big on fruits.

Pizza may qualify as the all-time favorite snack of America, followed closely by burgers and other fast food. There is a reason why most fast food restaurants are successful in America and throughout the world.

It has also been established that the average American drinks about a gallon of soda every week. Even drinks that are supposed to have a low-calorie count end up being calorie-bombs because of the doctoring that takes place. For instance, black coffee is low on calorie, but not so if it has milk and ice cream and sugar all over it.

Summary

The first-world economies are not alone in facing the crisis of obesity. It has emerged that people in poor countries are battling obesity too. Obesity-related deaths are on the rise. In 2017, the figures were especially shocking, for they'd surpassed the death count of terrorist attacks, accidents, and Alzheimer's combined. One of the corrective measures that the US government is considering to undertake is tax increment on sugars. The chief reason why we are so fat is our poor diets. Our foods are laden with sugars and fats, and it doesn't help that our lifestyles allow us to expend only a small amount of energy, which leads to fat accumulation and consequent weight gain. The average man requires around 2500 calories for his body to act optimally whereas the average woman requires 2000 calories. The top five daily sources of calories for Americans include desserts, bread, chicken, soda, and alcohol.

Chapter 3: Benefits of Fasting

Improved Insulin Sensitivity

Insulin sensitivity refers to how positively or negatively your body cells respond to insulin. If you have a high insulin sensitivity, you will need less amount of insulin to convert the sugars in your blood into energy, whereas someone with low insulin sensitivity would need a significantly larger amount of insulin.

Low insulin sensitivity is characterized by increased blood sugar levels. In other words, the insulin produced by the body is underutilized when converting sugars into energy. Low insulin sensitivity may make you vulnerable to ailments such as cancer, heart disease, type 2 diabetes, stroke, and dementia.

Ailments and bad moods are the general causes of low insulin sensitivity. However, high insulin sensitivity is restored once the ailments and bad moods are over.

Fasting is shown to have a positive effect on insulin sensitivity, enhancing your body to use small amounts of insulin to convert blood sugar into energy.

Improved insulin sensitivity has a great impact on health: leveling up physiological functions and fighting off common symptoms of ailments like lightheadedness and lethargy.

To increase insulin sensitivity, here are some of the best practices: perform physical activities, lose weight, consume foods that are high in fiber and low in Glycemic load, improve your moods and alleviate depressed feelings, and finally, make sure to improve the quality of your sleep.

The rate of insulin sensitivity is also heavily dependent on lifestyle changes. For instance, if you take up sports and exercise, insulin sensitivity goes up, but if you become lazy and inactive, it goes down.

- **Increased Leptin Sensitivity**

Leptin is the hormone that determines whether you're experiencing hunger or full. This hormone plays a critical role in weight loss and health management, and if your body grows insensitive to it, you become susceptible to some ailments. Understanding the role of leptin in your body is critical as it goes into helping you improve your health regimen.

Whenever this hormone is secreted by the fat cells, the brain takes notice, and it tries to determine whether you are in need of food or are actually full. Leptin needs to work as normally as possible else you will receive an inaccurate signal that will cause you to either overfeed or starve yourself.

Low leptin sensitivity induces obesity. This condition is normally witnessed in people with high levels of insulin. The excessive sugars in blood are carried off by insulin into fat cells, but when there is an insulin overload, a communication crash is triggered between fat cells and the brain. This condition induces low leptin sensitivity. When this happens, your brain is unable to tell the exact amount of leptin in your blood, and as such it misleads you. Low leptin sensitivity causes the brain to continue sending out the hunger signal even after you are full. This causes you to eat more than you should and, given time, leads to chronic weight gain.

Fasting has been shown to increase leptin sensitivity, a state that allows the brain to be precise in determining blood leptin quantities, and ensures that the accurate signal is transmitted to control your eating habits.

- **Normalized Ghrelin Levels**

Known as the "hunger hormone," ghrelin is instrumental in regulating both appetite and the rate of energy distribution into body cells.

Increased levels of ghrelin cause the brain to trigger hunger pangs and secrete gastric acids as the body anticipates you to consume food.

It is also important to note that both ghrelin and leptin receptors are located on the same group of brain cells, even though these hormones play contrasting roles, i.e., ghrelin being the hunger hormone, and leptin the satiety hormone.

The primary role of ghrelin is to increase appetite and see to it that the body has a larger fat reservoir. So, high ghrelin levels in your blood will result in you wanting to eat more food and, in some cases, particular foods like cake or fries or chocolate.

People who have low ghrelin levels will not eat enough amounts of food and are thus vulnerable to diseases caused by underfeeding. As a corrective measure, such people should receive shots of ghrelin to restore accurate hunger signals in their bodies.

Studies show that obese people suffer from a disconnection between their brains and ghrelin cells, so the blood ghrelin levels go through the roof, which makes these people be in a state of perpetual hunger. So, these obese people respond to their hunger pangs by indulging in their foods of choice, and thus the chronic weight gain becomes hard to manage.

It has been proven that fasting has a positive effect on ghrelin levels. Fasting streamlines the faulty communication between the brain receptors and ghrelin cells. When this is corrected, the brain starts to send out accurate hunger signals, discouraging you from eating more than you should.

- **Increased Lifespan And Slow Aging**

A study by Harvard researchers demonstrated that intermittent fasting led to an increased lifespan and the slowing down of the aging process. These findings were largely hinged on the cell-replenishing effects of fasting and flushing out of toxins.

The average person puts their digestive system under constant load because they're only a short moment away from their next meal. And given the fact that most foods are bacteria-laden, the immune system becomes strained with all the wars that it must be involved in. This makes the body cells prone to accelerated demise. But what happens when you go on a fast?

The energy that would have previously gone into digesting food is used to flush out toxins from the body instead. Also, it has been observed that body cells are strengthened during a fast, which makes physiological functions a bit more robust.

Fasting also enhances the creation of new neural pathways and regeneration of brain cells. This goes towards optimizing the functions of your brain. And, as we know, an energetic brain makes for a "youthful" life.

When you are on a fast, the blood sugar levels are generally down. The skin responds favorably to low blood sugar levels by improving elasticity and keeping wrinkles at bay. A high blood sugar level is notorious for making you ashy and wrinkly.

Fasting may increase your lifespan even from an indirect perspective. For instance, fasting may develop your sense of self-control, improve your discipline, and even increase your creativity. These immaterial resources are very necessary for surviving in the real world.

- **Improved Brain Function**

Fasting triggers the body to destroy its weak cells in a process known as autophagy. One of the main benefits of autophagy is reducing inflammation. Also, autophagy makes way for new and healthy body cells. Autophagy promotes neurogenesis, which is the creation of new brain cells.

Fasting allows the body to deplete the sugars in the blood, and since the body must continue to operate lest it shuts down, the body turns to an alternative energy source: fats. Through the aid of the liver, ketone bodies are produced to supply energy to the brain. Ketone bodies are a much cleaner and reliable source of energy than carbohydrates. Ketone bodies are known to tone down the effects of inflammatory diseases like arthritis.

Fasting promotes high insulin sensitivity. In this way, the body uses less insulin to convert sugars into energy. High insulin sensitivity means that the body will send out accurate signals when it comes to informing the host of either hunger or satiation.

Fasting enhances the production of BDNF (Brain-Derived Neurotrophic Factor), which a plays a critical part in improving neuroplasticity. And thus more resources are committed to the functions of the brain. BDNF is responsible for augmenting areas like memory, learning, and emotions.

Fasting supercharges your mind. It does so through facilitating the creation of new mitochondria. And since mitochondria are the power plants of our bodies, the energy output goes up. This increase in energy and resources causes the brain to function at a much higher level and yields perfect results.

- **Improved Strength And Agility**

When you think of a person that is considered strong and agile, your mind might conceive a well-muscled individual with veins bulging out their neck. Strength and agility come down to practice and more practice. The easiest way to develop agility and strength is obviously through physical training and sticking to a routine until your body adapts.

You must practice every day to be as strong and agile as you'd want to be. Also, you must take particular care over your dietary habits. Professional athletes stick to a diet that has been approved by their doctors for a reason. When it comes to developing strength and agility, nothing matches the combination of exercise and a flawless diet.

But besides fulfilling these two requirements, fasting, too, has its place. Did you know that you can amplify your strength and agility through fasting?

Fasting provokes the body to secrete the Human Growth Hormone. This hormone enhances organ development and even muscle growth. So when you fast, the HGH hormone might be secreted, and it will amplify the effects of your exercise and diet regimen, making you many times stronger and agile.

Fasting will promote the renewal of your body cells and thus lessen the effects of inflammation. When you perform physical exercises, you're basically injuring and damaging your body cells. So, when you fast, you'll allow your body to destroy its weak cells, and make room for new body cells through biogenesis.

Additionally, fasting will go a long way toward improving your motor skills, making you walk with the grace of a cat, with your body parts flexible.

- **Improved Immune System**

The immune system is responsible for defending your body against organisms that are disease vectors. When a foreign organism enters your body, and the body considers it harmful, the immune system immediately comes into action.

Some of the methods suggested for improving the immune system include having a balanced diet, quality sleep, improving your mental health, and taking physical exercises.

Fasting is an understated method of boosting your immune system.

In a research conducted by scientists at the University of Southern California, it emerged that fasting enhanced the rejuvenation of the immune system. Specifically, new white blood cells were formed, strengthening the body's defense system.

The regeneration of the immune system is especially beneficial to people who have a weak body defense mechanism—namely, the elderly, and the sick. This could probably be the reason why an animal in the wild responds to illness by abstaining from food.

In the same study, it was shown that there is a direct correlation between fasting and diminished radical elements in the body. Cell biogenesis was responsible for eradicating inflammation. And moreover, a replenished immune system discouraged the growth of cancer cells.

Depending on how long you observe a fast, the body will, at one point, run out of sugars, and then it will turn to your fat reservoirs to provide energy for its many physiological functions. Fats make for a much cleaner and stable and resourceful energy source than sugars ever will.

So, relying on this fat-energy, the immune system tends to function at a most optimal level.

- **Optimized Physiological Functions**

These are some of the body's physiological functions: sweating, bowel movement, temperature regulation, urinating, and stimuli response.

In a healthy person, all physiological functions should be seamless, but that cannot be said for most of us because our lifestyles get in the way.

So, the next time you rush to the bathroom intending to take a number two only to wind up spending half an hour there, you might want to take a close look at what you are eating.

Fasting is a great method of optimizing your physiological functions. When you observe a normal eating schedule, your body is under constant strain to keep digesting food—a resource-intensive process. But when you go on a fast, the energy that would have been used for digesting food will now be channeled into other critical functions. For instance, the body may now start ridding itself of radicals that promote indigestion, or amp up the blood circulation system, or even devote energy toward enhancing mental clarity, with the result being optimized physiological functions.

With more resources freed up from the strain of digestion, physiological processes will continue seamlessly, and once the glycogen in the blood is over, the body will continue to power physiological functions with energy acquired from fat cells.

The cellular repair benefits attached to fasting enables your body to perform its functions way better. Fasting reduces oxidative stress, which is a key accelerator of aging. In this way, fasting helps restore the youthfulness of your body cells, and the cells are very much optimized for performance.

- **Improved Cardiovascular Health**

When we talk about cardiovascular health, we are essentially talking about the state of the heart, and specifically, its performance in blood circulation.

Factors that improve the condition of your heart include a balanced diet, improved emotional and mental state, quality sleep, and living in a good environment. When cardiovascular health is compromised, it might lead to fatal consequences.

Researchers have long established that fasting improves cardiovascular health.

One of the outcomes of fasting is cholesterol reduction. The lesser cholesterol you have in your blood, the more seamless the movement of blood through your body. Complications are minimal or nonexistent. Thus your heart will be in a great condition.

Fasting also plays a critical role in toning down diabetes. The average diabetic tends to have low insulin sensitivity. For that reason, they need more insulin than is necessary to convert sugars into energy. It puts a strain on body organs and especially the pancreas. This might cause a trickle-down complication that goes back to the heart.

When the body enters fasting mode, it starts using up the stored energy to fulfill other important physiological functions such as blood circulation, in this way boosting the effectiveness of the heart.

Fasting helps you tap into your "higher state." The effects of matured spiritual energy and peaceful inner self cannot be gainsaid. Someone who's at peace with both himself and the universe is bound to develop a very healthy heart, as opposed to one who's constantly bitter, and one who feels as though he's drowning in a bottomless pit.

• **Low Blood Pressure**

People who have a high blood pressure are at risk of damaging not only their heart but their arteries too. When the pressure of the blood flowing in your arteries is high over a long period of time, it is bound to damage the cells of your arteries, and in the worst case scenario, it might trigger a rupture, and cause internal bleeding. High blood pressure puts you at risk of heart failure. Your heart might overwork itself and slowly start wearing out, eventually grinding to a halt.

In people with high blood pressure, a bigger-than-normal left heart is common, and the explanation is that their left heart struggles to maintain the cardiovascular output. So it starts bulking up and eventually creates a disrupting effect on your paired organ. Another risk associated with high blood pressure is coronary disease. This ailment causes your arteries to thin out to the point that it becomes a struggle for blood to flow into your heart. The dangers of coronary disease include arrhythmia, heart failure, and chest pain.

I started by mentioning the risks of high blood pressure because observing a fast normalizes your blood pressure. With a normal blood pressure, you can reverse these risks. Also, normal blood pressure improves the sensitivity of various hormones like ghrelin and leptin, eliminating the communication gap between brain receptors and body cells.

The low blood pressure induced by fasting causes you to have improved motor skills. It is common to hear people admit that fasting makes them feel light and flexible.

- **Decreased Inflammation**

Inflammation is an indication that the body is fighting against an infectious organism. It causes the affected parts to appear red and swollen.

Many diseases that plague us today are rooted in inflammation, and by the look of things, inflammation will be stuck with us for longer than we imagine.

The role of inflammation in mental health cannot be understated. Inflammation is to blame for bad moods, depression, and social anxiety.

The good news though is that fasting can reduce inflammation. Fasting has been shown to be effective in treating mental problems that are rooted in inflammation and as well as safeguarding neural pathways.

Individuals who have incorporated fasting into their lives are much less likely to suffer breakdowns and bad moods than people who don't fast at all.

Asthma, a lung infection, also has an inflammatory background. What's interesting is that fasting alleviates the symptoms of asthma.

The level of hormone sensitivity determines absorption rates of various elements into body cells. For instance, low insulin sensitivity worsens the rate of conversion of sugar into energy. Fasting improves insulin sensitivity, and thus more sugars can be converted into energy.

Fasting enhances the brain to form new pathways when new information is discovered. In this way, your memory power receives a boost, and you are better placed to handle stress and bad thoughts.

Fasting is very efficient in alleviating gut inflammation. Constant fasting promotes healthy gut flora which makes for great bowel movements.

Fasting is a great means of reducing heart inflammation, too. It does so through stabilizing blood pressure and fighting off radical elements.

- **Improved Skin Care**

Most of us are very self-conscious about how we look to the world. Bad skin, acne, and other skin ailments can be a real bother. Fasting has numerous benefits when it comes to improving your skin health, and it is said that fasting bestows a glow on your face. Experts claim that skin ailments develop as a result of terrible stomach environments and that there is a correlation between gut health and skin quality. Fasting promotes the development of gut flora. In this way, your gut health is improved, resulting in improved skin.

When you are on a fast and are taking water, you will eliminate toxins from your body. The condition of your skin improves because the skin cells are free of harmful substances. Many people who previously suffered from a bad skin condition and had tried almost every treatment with no success have admitted that fasting was the only thing that worked.

Another benefit of fasting is that it slows down the aging process. The water consumed during the fast goes to flush out toxins, consequently reducing the effects of old age on your skin. Fasting also promotes low blood sugar. Low blood sugar promotes optimized physiological processes and, as a result, toning down the effects of aging.

When you go on a fast, the body allocates energy to areas that might have previously been overlooked. So, your bad skin condition may be treated with the stored up energy, and considering that the energy produced from fat is more stable and resourceful; your skin health will improve.

- **Autophagy**

This is the process whereby the body rids itself of weakened and damaged cells. Autophagy is triggered by dry fasting. The body simply "eats" the weakened cells to provide water to the healthy cells. Eliminated cells are usually weak and damaged. And their absence creates room for new cells that are obviously going to be powerful.

Autophagy has been shown to have many benefits, and they include:

- **Slowing down aging effects**

The formation of wrinkles and body deterioration are some of the effects of aging. However, thanks to autophagy, these effects can be reversed, since the body will destroy its old and weakened cells and replace them with new cells.

- **Reducing inflammation**

Inflammation is responsible for many diseases affecting us today, but thanks to autophagy, the cells that have been affected by inflammation are consumed, giving room for new cells.

- **Conserving energy**

Autophagy elevates the body into a state of energy conservation. In this way, your body can utilize resources in a most careful manner.

- **Fighting infections**

The destruction of old and weak body cells creates room for fresh and powerful body cells. In that vein, old and weakened white blood cells are destroyed, and then new powerful white blood cells are formed. These new white new blood cells fortify the immune system.

- **Improving motor skills**

Autophagy plays a critical role in improving the motor skills of an individual. This goes toward boosting the strength and agility of a person. Energy drawn from the weak and damaged cells is way more resourceful than the energy drawn from sugars.

Summary

There are numerous benefits attached to fasting. One of them is increased insulin sensitivity. When the insulin sensitivity goes up, insulin resistance drops, and the body is now able to use less insulin to convert sugars into energy. Another benefit of fasting is improved leptin sensitivity. The leptin hormone is known as the satiation hormone, and it is responsible for alerting you when you are full. An improved ghrelin level is another benefit of fasting. The ghrelin hormone is known as the hunger hormone. It induces hunger pangs so that you may feed. Fasting lengthens your existence. This is largely because of neuroregeneration of cells and flushing out toxins. Fasting improves brain function, strengthens your body and boosts agility, strengthens your immune system, optimizes your physiological functions, improves cardiovascular health, lowers blood pressure, reduces inflammation, improves your skin, and promotes autophagy. As researchers carry out new experiments, more benefits of fasting are being uncovered.

Chapter 4: Myths and Dangers of Fasting

Long-Held Myths and Misconceptions about Fasting

Fasting has gained widespread acceptance across the world. More people who are seeking to improve their health through alternative means are turning to fasting. As you might expect, the field has been marred with conspiracies, lies, half-truths, and outright ignorance. Some of the long-held myths and misconceptions about fasting include:

Fasting makes you overeat. This myth hinges on the idea that after observing a fast, an individual is bound to be so hungry that they will consume more food to compensate for the period they'd abstained from food.

The brain requires a steady supply of sugars. Some people say that the brain cannot operate normally in the absence of sugars. These people believe that the brain uses sugars alone to power its activities and any other source of energy would not be compatible. So when you fast, you'd be risking shutting down your brain functions.

Skipping breakfast will make you fat. Some people seem to treat breakfast as though it were an unexplained mystery of the Earth. They say breakfast is special. Anyone who misses breakfast cannot possibly have a healthy life. They say that if you skip breakfast, you will be under a heavy spell of cravings, and finally give in to unhealthy foods.

Fasting promotes eating disorders. Some people seem to think that fasting is the stepping stone for disorders like bulimia and anorexia. They complain that once you see the effects of fasting, you might want to "amplify" the effects which might make you susceptible to an eating disorder like anorexia.

Busting Myths Associated with Fasting

Fasting will make you overeat. This is partly true. However, it is important to note that most people fall into the temptation of overeating because of their lack of discipline and not necessarily because of unrealistic demands of fasting. If you're fasting the proper way, no temptation is big enough to lead you astray, and after all, the temptation exists to test whether you're really disciplined.

The brain requires a steady supply of sugars. This myth perpetuates the notion that we should consume carbohydrates every now and again to keep the brain in working condition. Also, this myth suggests that the brain can only use energy derived from sugars and not energy derived from fats. When you go on a fast, and your body uses up all the glycogen, your liver produces ketone bodies that are passed on to your brain to act as an energy source.

Skipping breakfast will make you fat. There is nothing special about breakfast. You can decide to skip breakfast and adhere to your schedule and be able to get desired results. It's true that skipping breakfast will cause you to be tempted by cravings, but you're not supposed to give in, and in that case, you become the problem. Skipping breakfast will not make you fat. What will make you fat is you pouring more calories into your body than you will spend.

Fasting promotes eating disorders. If you have a goal in mind, you are supposed to stay focused on that goal. The idea that an individual would plunge into the world of eating disorders simply because they want to amplify the results of fasting sounds like weakness on the part of the individual and not a fault of the practice itself.

Dangers of Fasting

Just as with most things in life, there's both a positive and negative side to fasting. Most of these problems are amplified in people who either fast in the wrong way or people who clearly shouldn't be fasting.

So let's explore some of the risks that are attached to fasting.

- **Dehydration**

Chances are, you will suffer dehydration while observing a fast, and drinking regular cups of water won't make the situation any better. Well, this is because most of your water intake comes from the foods that you consume daily. When dehydration kicks in, you are bound to experience nausea, headaches, constipation, and dizziness.

- **Orthostatic Hypotension**

This is common in people who drink water during their fasts. Orthostatic Hypotension causes your body to react unfavorably when you move around. For instance, when you stand on your feet and walk around, you might experience dizziness and feel as though you're at the verge of blowing up into smithereens. Other symptoms include temporary mental blindness, lightheadedness, and vision problems. These symptoms make it hard for you to function in activities that demand precision and focus, e.g., driving.

- **Worsened medical conditions**

People who fast while they are sick put themselves at risk of worsening their condition. The fast may amplify the symptoms of their diseases. People with the following ailments should first seek doctor's approval before getting into fasting: gout, type 2 diabetes, chronic kidney disease, eating disorders, and heartburn.

- **Increased stress**

The habit of skipping meals might lead to increased stress. The body might respond to hunger by increasing the hormone cortisol which is responsible for high-stress levels. And when you are in a stressed mental state, it becomes difficult to function in your day to day life.

Summary

Although fasting has a lot of benefits, there is a dark side to it too, but the negative effects can be minimized or eliminated altogether when a professional is involved. Dehydration is one of the negative effects. Besides providing nutrients to the body, food is also an important source of water. So when you fail to correct this gap by drinking a lot more water, your body will fall into a state of dehydration. Orthostatic hypotension is another danger. This illness makes you feel dizzy and lightheaded, and so it makes it difficult for you to function in an activity that demands your focus and stamina. Fasting may amplify the symptoms of your disease depending on your age and the stage of your disease. For instance, people who suffer from illnesses like gout, diabetes, eating disorders, and heartburn should first seek the doctor's approval before going on a fast. Moreover, fasting may lead to an increase in stress levels.

Chapter 5: Safety, Side Effects, and Warning

The Safest and Enlightened Way of Fasting

As the subject of fasting becomes popular, more people are stating their opinions on it, and as you might expect, some people are for it, and others are against it.

The best approach toward fasting is not set in stone, but it is rather determined by factors such as your age and health status.

Before you get into fasting, there are some critical balances you need to consider first. One of them is your experience. If you have never attempted a fast before, then it is a bad idea to go straight into a 48-hour fast, because you are likely to water down the effects. As a beginner, you must always start with lighter fasts and build your way up into extended fasts. You could begin by skipping one meal, then two meals, and finally the whole day.

Another important metric when it comes to determining the appropriate space between your eating windows is your health status. For instance, you cannot be a sufferer of late-stage malaria and yet go on a fast, because it might create a multiplying effect on your symptoms. People who are malnourished or have eating disorders might want to find other ways of improving their health apart from fasting.

An essential thing to note is that we are not all alike. My body's response to a fast is not going to be the exact response of yours. Knowing this, always listen to your body. Sometimes, a water-fast might trigger a throat infection and make your throat swollen. In such a situation, it would be prudent to suspend the fast and take care of your throat, as opposed to sticking to your guns.

Side Effects of Fasting

Fasting might upset the physiological functions of a body. This explains the side effects that crop up when you go on a fast. It is also important to note that most of these side effects subside as your body grows accustomed to the fast.

- **Cravings**

Top on the list is cravings. When you go on a fast, the immediate response by the body is to elevate the "hunger hormone" and so, you will start craving for sweet unhealthy foods. If you are not the disciplined type, this is a huge pitfall that could negate the effects of your fast.

- **Headaches**

Headaches, too, are a side effect of fasting. Most people who are new to fasting are bound to experience a headache. One of the explanations for headaches is that it is the brain's response to a shift from relying on carbohydrates to ketone bodies as the alternative energy source. Regular consumption of water might mitigate the headache or eliminate it altogether.

- **Low energy**

Another side effect is low energy. When you fast, the body might interpret it as starving, and its first response will be conserving energy. So, there will be less energy for physiological functions. In this way, you will start feeling less energetic than before.

- **Irritability**

Irritability is also a side effect. Studies show that people who are new to fasting are bound to have foul moods as their body increases stress hormones and hunger hormones. However, if they can persist, the irritability will eventually go away, and make room for a happy mood as the body switches to its fat stores for energy.

Types of People That Should Not Fast

The ideal person to go on a fast is a healthy person. People with certain medical conditions may still go on a fast, but it is always prudent to seek the guidance of a medical professional. We have previously stated that fasting strengthens the immune system. So is it contradicting to discourage fasting when one is sick? No! You may fast but preferably under the instruction and supervision of a medical professional. However, there are cases when it is inappropriate to fast.

Infants and children. Putting kids on a fast is just wrong. Their bodies are not fully developed yet to withstand periods of hunger. Fasting would do them more damage than good. For instance, it might mess with their metabolism and have a negative impact on their growth curve.

Hypoglycemics. People with hypoglycemia have extremely low levels of blood sugar. Their bodies need a constant stream of sugars to sustain normal functions lest severe illnesses take reign. For that reason, hypoglycemics should not fast.

Pregnant and nursing women. These women need a lot of energy because their young ones are dependent on them. So, pregnant women and nursing women are encouraged to keep their blood sugar steady.

The malnourished. People who are underweight and malnourished should stay away from fasting. To start with, their bodies don't have sufficient fat. So, when they go on a fast, their body will destroy its cells in search of nutrients. Over time, the results could be fatal.

People with heartburn. People who experience severe heartburn should not fast. This is because heartburn is a very distressing thing and there is no guarantee it will subside even when your body adapts to fasting. So, it is better to stay clear.

Impaired immune system. Fasting may have the ability to renew the strength and utility of your immune system. But when we are talking about an impaired immune system where most of the white blood cells are hanging on a thin blade, then fasting cannot be of help. Such a person would be better off sticking to a healthy diet.

Other classes of people that shouldn't fast include those recovering from surgeries, people with eating disorders, depressed souls, and people with extreme heart disease.

Summary
For purposes of safety, always ensure that your body is prepared to withstand the effects of fasting. You may prepare by evaluating your health status, experience, and developing a great sense of self-awareness. Fasting may have its numerous benefits, but there is also a negative side to it because fasting comes with unpleasant side effects. The good thing though is that most of these side effects tend to subside once the body grows accustomed to your fasting routine. One of the side effects of fasting is getting a headache. A headache is triggered by the brain's adjustment from relying on carbohydrates as an energy source and switching to ketone bodies. It may be mitigated through constant consumption of water. Another side effect is cravings. Your body makes you want to eat fast foods very badly. Fasting may also make you irritable, but it is for only a short time and then a happy mood sets in. Fasting also makes you feel less energetic, which can be uninspiring. These are some of the people that shouldn't fast: hypoglycemics, infants, children, pregnant women, nursing women, the malnourished, people with extreme ailments, and those recovering from surgeries.

Part 2: Types of Fasting and How to Fast

Chapter 6: Intermittent Fasting

What Is Intermittent Fasting?

Nowadays, intermittent fasting is one of the most talked about practices in health improvement domains. Basically, intermittent fasting is about creating a routine where you eat only after a set period of time. Intermittent fasting has been shown to have numerous benefits such as improving motor skills, developing willpower, and brain functions. Most people are turning to the practice to achieve their health goals—specifically, weight loss.

The most common way of performing an intermittent fast is by skipping meals. In the beginning, you may decide to skip one of the main meals, and when your body adapts to two meals a day, you may then elevate to just one meal per day. During the fast, you are not supposed to partake of any food, but it is okay to drink water and other low-calorie drinks like black coffee or black tea.

Intermittent fasting allows you to indulge in the foods of your choice, but there's emphasis on avoiding foods that are traditionally bad for your health. The main thing is to give your body time to process food between your eating windows.

Polls answered by people who have adopted this lifestyle indicate that most of them are happy with the results. Intermittent fasting is a very effective means of weight loss as it improves the metabolic rate of the body, as well as triggers cell autophagy. The good thing about intermittent fasting is that it allows you to partake of your favorite foods without making you feel guilty, which is a contrast to fad diets that insist on eating things like raw food and plant-based foods.

How to Practice Intermittent Fasting

There are a couple of ways to practice intermittent fasting. These are the three most popular ways:

- **The 16/8 method**

In this method, you are supposed to fast for 16 hours. Your eating window is restricted to eight hours every day. For instance, you might choose to only eat between twelve noon and eight in the evening.

- **Eat-Stop-Eat**

This fast involves irregular abstinence from food for a full 24 hours. You might decide to practice this once or twice every week. But when you fast, you must wait for 24 hours to pass before you indulge in the next meal. The eat-stop-eat method is very effective in not only weight loss but also in flushing out toxins from the body over the 24 hours you abstained from food.

- **The 5:2 Diet**

This type of intermittent fasting demands that you devote two days every week where you'll consume not more than 600 calories. Considering that the daily caloric requirement for the average person is 2000–2500, this type of fast will create a caloric deficit, and there's going to be weight loss as the body taps into its fat reservoirs for energy.

- **Alternate-Day Fasting**

This type of fasting requires that you skip one day and fast the next day. Depending on the intensity you want, you might choose to have a zero calorie intake or restrict your calorie intake to not more than 600. Alternate-day fasting is suitable for people who have experience with fasting and only want to escalate to amplify the benefits. A newbie should start with small fasts.

Pros and Cons of Intermittent Fasting

Intermittent fasting helps you save up on weekly food costs. That's a big advantage in these hard economic times. Food can be a very expensive affair especially if you eat out.

Intermittent fasting allows you to focus on your life goals. The energy that would have gone into looking for or preparing your next meal is used up to attain your important goals. Intermittent fasting has the potential to improve your emotional being and reduce anxiety—all of which make your life more stress-free.

Intermittent fasting is doable and safe. This means that it is free of complications and there's nothing to hold back anyone that wants to go into it. This is unlike other methods of weight loss like fad diets where some foods might be hard to access or expensive, or you dislike them.

Intermittent fasting improves the body's sensitivity to insulin, and by extension, it improves the metabolic rate of your body.

Moving on to the cons—the biggest disadvantage of intermittent fasting is the social dynamics. For instance, you might be out with friends when they decide to "pop in a joint" and then it's going to be strange to explain that you won't eat or maybe you'll defy your fasting routine and eat anyway, in which case you have cheated yourself.

Intermittent fasting doesn't seem to have a coherent and stable method. There are so many variations that dilute the philosophy of fasting. It almost feels like I can even come out with my style and popularize it. So, intermittent fasting lacks in originality.

Finding Your Ideal Intermittent Fasting Plan

The first and most important thing is to determine your health condition. If your body can permit you to indulge in intermittent fasting then, by all means, go ahead. If you are a beginner, you should start small, which means don't go from regular meals and start practicing 24-hour fasts.

That's counterproductive. Make sure you have some experience before you fast for an extended period of time.

You'll find that what works for someone won't necessarily work for everybody else. So what's one supposed to do? Test, test, test. At one point you will find a variation of the intermittent fast that will fit perfectly into your life. It's all about finding what really works for you and then committing to the routine.

In my experience, I have found the 16:8 to be the best. This type of intermittent fast requires that you abstain from food for 16 hours and then indulge for 8 hours. For most followers of this routine, they like to have their eating window between 12:00 PM and 20:00 PM. The 16-hour fast will be inclusive of sleep, which makes it less severe.

This method is extremely efficient in weight loss, and most people have reported success. However, you must stick to the routine for a while before you can see any results. Don't do it for just one day and climb on the weighing machine only to find that there are no changes and then give up.

To improve the success of fasting intermittently, stick to a balanced diet during your eating windows, and don't take the fast as an excuse for indulging in unhealthy foods.

Step-By-Step Process of Fasting For a Week

The first step is to certify that you are in perfect condition. Get an appointment with your doctor and perform a whole health analysis to get a clean bill of health. Remember to always start with a small fast and gradually build up.

- **Day one**

When you wake up, forgo breakfast and opt for a glass of water or black coffee. Then go on about your work as you normally do. Around noon, your eating window opens. Now you are free to indulge in the food of your choice, but make sure that they are nutritious foods because unhealthy foods will water down your efforts. Your eating window should close at 20:00 PM, and from 20:01 pm to 12:00 pm the next day, don't consume anything else besides water.

- **Day two**

On day two, your body should have started to protest over the sudden calorie reduction, and so you'll be likely experiencing an irritable mood, lightheadedness, and a small headache. When you wake up, no matter how strong the urge to eat might be, just push it back, and the only thing you should consume is water or black coffee. At noon, your eating window opens, and you're free to eat until 8 pm.

- **Day three**

When you wake up, take a glass of water or black coffee. Chances are that your body has started to adjust to the reduced daily caloric intake. It has switched to burning fats. At twelve noon, when your eating window opens, consume less food than you did yesterday and the day before, so that the body has even lesser calories to work with. The body should adapt to this pretty swiftly.

- **Day four**

In the morning, take a glass of water or black coffee and go about your business. When your eating window opens, eat as much food as you ate yesterday, but in the evening, resist the urge to drink anything.

- **Day five**

When you wake up, take a glass of water or black coffee. During your eating window, eat less food than you did previously. At night, resist the urge to drink water.

- **Day six**

When you wake up, resist the urge to drink water or even coffee. In your eating window, choose not to eat at all, and at night give in to the temptation and drink water or black coffee.

- **Day seven**

When you wake up, take a glass of water or black coffee. In your eating window, resume eating, but only take a small portion, and just before you close the eating window, eat again, except it should be a slightly larger meal than previously. Before you sleep, take another glass of water or black coffee. Fast till your next eating window, and then you may resume your normal eating habits. At this point, you will have lost weight and experienced a host of other benefits attached to intermittent fasting.

Summary

Intermittent fasting features a cycle of fasting interrupted by an eating window. Some of the methods of intermittent fasting include the 16:8, eat-stop-eat, 5:2, and alternate-day fasting. The best approach to intermittent fasting is context-based in the sense that only you can know what works for you. The most popular form of intermittent fasting is the 16:8. In this method, you fast for 16 hours and then an eating window of 8 hours. The biggest advantage of intermittent fasting is that it announces relief to your pocket. The "food budget" goes into other uses. The amount of time that it takes to prepare meals is a real hassle, but intermittent fasting frees up your time so you can be more productive. The entry barrier is nonexistent too. This means anyone can practice intermittent fasting because there are no barriers or things to buy—a stark contrast to other weight loss methods like fad diets that may be both inconveniencing and expensive.

Chapter 7: Longer Periods of Fasting

What is Fasting for Longer Periods?

Fasting for longer periods is reserved for people who have a bit of experience with fasting. A newbie shouldn't get into it.

It is basically desisting from food for not less than 24 hours, but not more than, say, 48 hours. You may increase the success of the fast by making it a dry fast. In a dry fast, you won't have the luxury of drinking water or any other low-calorie drink like black coffee.

Fasting for longer periods requires that you prepare emotionally, mentally, and physically. The buildup to your fast is an especially important part. Your food consumption should be minimal.

Fasting for a longer period helps you achieve much more results because the body will be subjected to an increased level of strain.

However, you must take care to know when to stop. In some instances, the body might rebel by either catching an infection or shutting down critical functions, and in such times it is prudent to call off the fast.

During longer fasts, you should abstain from strenuous exercises, because the body will be in a state of energy conservation, and the available energy is purposed for physiological functions.

With the wrong approach, long fasts might become disastrous. That's why it is always important to seek clearance from your doctor first before you go into the fast. And to flush out toxins, ensure you have a steady intake of water.

It is estimated that weight loss in longer fasts averages around one to two pounds every day.

How to Fast for Longer Periods

The main reason that people go into longer fasts is to obviously lose weight. But you might want to fast to reach other purposes such as flushing toxins from your body or heightening your mental capabilities. Also, a longer fast is recommended if you are going into a surgery.

The response to a fast is different for everyone. If it is your first time, please take great care by getting medical clearance.

As your fast approaches, you might want to minimize your food consumption to get used to managing hunger.

Next, you should clear away items that might ruin your focus or tempt you to backslide. You might want to give your kitchen a total makeover by, for instance, clearing away the bad food. It is much easier to manage cravings when they are out of sight than when they are within easy reach.

Always start small. Before you deprive yourself food for over 24 hours, you should first get a taste of what food deprivation for 8 hours feels like, and if you can handle that, then you're ready to step up your game. While you fast, you should be very aware of the ranges of effects that your body experiences. You might feel dizzy, lightheaded, sleepy, or distressed, and these are okay reactions. Things that are not okay are infections and prolonged aches of body parts. If your body responds to fasting unfavorably, you should stop the fast.

Pros and Cons of Fasting for Longer Periods

If you have always been motivated to clear away the stubborn fat in your body, but have never found an efficient method, then the answer is to fast for a longer period.

When you go on a longer fast, the body uses up all glycogen in the first 24 hours, and then it switches to burning fats. A longer fast guarantees quick weight loss.

A longer fast saves you money. Food is an expensive affair, especially if you eat out. With a longer fast, it means you are staying away from food, and are thus saving on food costs.

Besides the benefit of optimizing your health, a longer fast will strengthen both your willpower and mental sharpness, which are two necessary factors in attaining success.

Fasting for a longer period helps you appreciate the taste of food. By the time you're done fasting, you'll want to indulge your appetite, and food will suddenly taste so sweet. The scarcity factor elevates the value of food.

A longer fast has cons, too. One of the biggest cons is the strain that it puts on your body. When your body goes from relying on glycogen into fats as a source of energy, nasty side effects are bound to come up—for instance, headaches, nausea, and lightheadedness.

Another con is that fasting for a longer period might open you up to disease. As much as fasting renews your immune system, your body still needs robust energy to function optimally. Fasting puts your body into a state of conserving energy which makes it easy for disease to attack.

Step-By-Step Process of Fasting for Longer Periods

When you decide to go on a fast for a longer period, you must realize that you are signing up for a real challenge. The body's immediate response to a fast is raising the hunger hormone to alert you to look for food. Now, fighting off that urge takes a lot of willpower. In some regard, it's why fasting might be considered a test of discipline because not so many people can withstand it.

So here's the step-by-step process of going on a fast for longer periods:

Preparation

The first major thing is to ensure that your body is in a condition that will allow you to fast, without any complications. In other words, consult your doctor for a checkup.

Reduce your food intake in the days leading up to your fast so that your body can get accustomed to staying without food. Once your body is familiar with the feeling of food deprivation, you are ready to move forward.

In the morning of your fast, drink lots of water. It is critical for flushing out toxins and reducing stomach acidity when your stomach secretes acids in anticipation of food. Your water intake should be regular and spread out through the day.

Rather than lying down and wearing a look of self-pity, just go on about your work as you normally would, provided it is not a very focus-oriented job like performing surgeries.

You should stay the whole day without food and then go to bed. On the following morning, your hunger pangs will be even more amplified, at which point you are to mitigate the hunger with a drink of water and then maintain the fast for another 24 hours. 48 hours are enough for a longer fast, and the weight loss should be dramatic. After the fast, don't immediately go back to eating heavy amounts of food, but rather ease your way into a lighter diet.

Chapter 8: Extended Fasting

How to Fast for Extended Periods

Fasting for an extended period is an extreme form of fasting that demands you abstain from food from anywhere between three days to seven days. If you can deny yourself food for more than three days, you should be proud of yourself, because not so many people have that kind of determination.

Fasting for an extended period of time amplifies the results of a longer fast. When you go for an extended period of time without food, you will allow yourself to experience a range of different feelings. At the initial stage there is distress, and towards the end your feelings become tranquil.

Considering that this is an especially long fast, you are supposed to take a very keen listen to the response by your body. If your body sends out the message that it is under massive strain, now it's time to stop the fast. Cases where it's appropriate to stop include developing stomach ulcers, throat infection, and loss of consciousness.

You should eat lighter meals as you approach the start of your fast. During the fast, your water intake should be regular. When you complete the fast, the transition to your normal eating life should be slow and gradual, starting with lighter meals.

Fasting for an extended period has the biggest potential of going wrong. The prolonged food deprivation in itself may do more good than harm. There is also the possibility of slightly altering your body's physiological functions. Still, the benefits of an extended fast outweigh the negatives.

Pros and Cons of Fasting for Extended Periods

The biggest advantage of fasting for an extended period of time is the discipline it instills in you. When you go for a prolonged period without eating food, your body will respond by increasing hunger pangs. It takes extreme willpower to keep going. This experience can help you build your self-control and discipline in real life.

An extended fast is very effective in banishing stubborn fat. Most people who are obese will tell you that they are trying to lose weight, but the fat is stubborn. Guess what, their methods are ineffective. However, if they had the will and courage to go on an extended fast, then they'd experience a rapid weight loss and reach their desired weight.

Extended fasting promotes a high rate of cell replenishing. When the body goes for days without food, it turns in on itself and begins to digest its cells—the weak and damaged cells—to provide nutrition for the healthy cells. The elimination of weak and damaged cells creates room for new and healthy ones.

The biggest disadvantage for an extended period of fasting is the risk of complications that you put your body into. Some complications might be instant whereas others may develop long after the fast. The biggest risk is catching an infection. If you're unlucky enough that you catch some disease in your fast, your immune system will be overwhelmed.

Another huge miss about extended fasting is the disconnect it encourages in your normal life. When you are fasting, you won't be able to share a meal with your friends or family, and that can be a big inconvenience. It can make people "talk."

Step-By-Step Process of Fasting for Extended Periods

When you get clearance from a medical professional, you should start by preparing for the extended fast. Ideally, if you are getting into an extended fast, you should have experience with either intermittent fasting, longer fasting or both. The more your body is familiar with food deprivation, the better the outcome.

On the start of your extended fast, you should consume only water or black coffee, and throughout the rest of the day, observe regular water consumption. It will aid in flushing out toxins and other harmful elements from your body.

During the fast, you should keep your normal work schedule, as opposed to being inactive, because inactivity will worsen your hunger pangs. The standard response to hunger pangs should be water consumption.

On the second day, first thing in the morning is to consume more water. This water is very critical in flushing out toxins and keeping your body cells hydrated as well as regulating autophagy. However, if you want to increase the success rate of the fast, you might consider eliminating water. One of the side effects of this type of fast is a dry mouth. A dry mouth has the potential of being very distressing. For purposes of safety, always hydrate yourself.

On the third day, wake up and consume water or black coffee. At this point, your body is subsisting on its fat reserves, and the weight loss is evident. Your body has potentially minimized hunger pangs to manageable levels. Keep yourself busy. Otherwise, inactivity will provoke hunger.

From the fourth day up until the seventh, keep the same routine. When you come to the end of your fast, realize that your body will be in starvation mode, so don't immediately consume large amounts of food. Instead, ease your way back into a normal eating schedule.

Chapter 9: The Eating Window

What is the Eating Window?

The eating window is the period of time that you are allowed to indulge in foods and one that precedes a period of fasting. The eating window comes around on a cycle, and you should adhere to it by only eating when the window opens and abstaining from food the rest of the time.

The hours are not set in stone. You are free to choose your eating window in a way that works for you. Most people who practice intermittent fasting seem to adhere to an eight-hour eating window followed by a sixteen-hour fast. Commonly, the eight-hour window opens at around 12:00 PM and goes all the way to 20:00 PM. During this time, you may indulge in your favorite foods. However, past 20:00 PM, you are supposed to observe the fast.

The 16:8 method of intermittent fasting appeals to many people because the 16 hours of fasting are inclusive of the bed-time. If you are not into waiting for sixteen hours before you partake of food, you may lessen the hours, so that you will have frequent eating windows between your fasts.

It is generally more fruitful to have a small eating window followed by a long period of fast.

It's also important to choose an eating window that optimizes your health. For instance, eating during the day is of much benefit than eating at night. This is because the body puts more calories to use during the day as opposed to while you are asleep. Also, adhere to a good diet, or else your gains will be neutralized by a bad diet.

What to Eat

The reason why intermittent fasting appeals to so many people is the nonexistent dietary rules common in alternative weight loss methods like fad diets. In intermittent fasting, you are free to eat the foods of your choice, and the main thing is to restrict your caloric intake.

You are free to consume the foods that delight you, but be careful not to fall in the pit of overcompensation. You are at risk of misleading yourself into consuming unhealthy foods during your eating window under the delusion that fasting will take care of it. Truth is, some of the fast foods we indulge are so calorie-laden that it would take a prolonged fast (not intermittent) to eliminate their fat from our bodies.

Limit your intake of red meat. As much as intermittent fasting is lenient when it comes to diet, it is widely known that red meat causes more harm than good. So, you might want to limit its intake or eliminate it altogether.

Fruits are a source of essential nutrients for the body. Always make sure to include fruits like bananas, avocados, and apples into your meals. Fruits help reduce inflammation and are critical in optimizing the physiological functions of the body.

Vegetables should be in your meals. People who claim that vegetables taste bad are just unimaginative cooks. Vegetables do taste good. And some of the health benefits of vegetable include strengthening your bones, stabilizing your blood sugar, boosting your brain health, and improving your digestive system.

Developing Discipline

It takes a lot of discipline to persevere through a fast. Think about it. The average person is accustomed to eating something every now and then. They cannot afford to hold back for even a couple more hours when lunch is due. The eating cycle never ends. And so a person who can decide to abstain from food and stick to their decision is a special kind of person—he/she is disciplined.

The biggest challenge when it comes to fasting for an extended period is to overcome the hunger pangs over the first few days. Your body floods you with the hunger hormone, pushing you to look for food. However, if you persevere through the first few days, your body will adjust to the food deprivation and switch to your stored fats as the alternative source of energy.

One of the things you must do to boost your self-control is to prepare your mind. When you have an idea of what to expect, the hunger will be more tolerable as opposed to if you're ignorant. Another thing to take into consideration is the weather. You don't want to fast during a cold season because fasting lowers your body temperature, and so you'll be hard-hit.

Another way of boosting your discipline is joining hands with people of the same goal. In this way, you can keep each other in check. When you are on a team or have a friend who practices fasting too, it will be easy to stick to your plan, as everybody will offer psycho-social support to everybody else. Sometimes, the difference between throwing in the towel and sticking to your guns is a kind word of encouragement.

Summary

The eating window is the period of time that you are allowed to indulge in foods and one that precedes a period of fasting. The eating window comes around on a cycle, and you should adhere to it by only eating when the window opens and abstaining from food the rest of the time. Intermittent fasting doesn't restrict the consumption of certain foods as is common for other weight loss methods such as fad diets. To boost the effectiveness of your fast, your diet should be balanced, which means it should include foods rich in minerals and vitamins. There also should be fruits and vegetables. Discipline is very important when it comes to fasting. It's what keeps you going when your body protests hunger. The most important step toward developing discipline is to first prepare mentally for the fast. Another way of developing discipline is by having a strong support system.

Part 3: Targeted Fasting for Your Body Type

Chapter 10: Fasting For Weight Loss

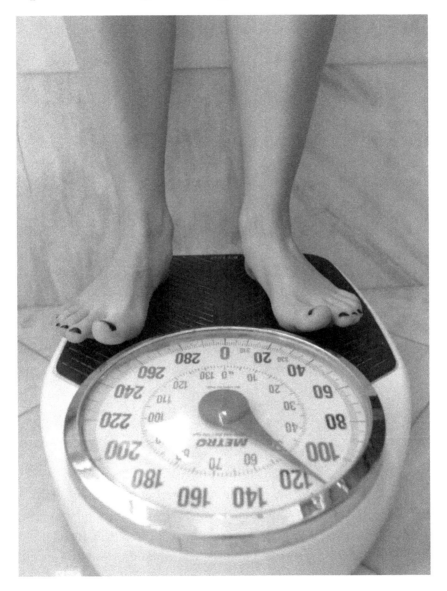

Why You'll Lose Weight through Fasting

Some of the methods of losing weight include fad diets, exercising, and supplements. However, these methods are not very effective, and in most cases, they cannot solve obesity on their own.

Fasting is easily the best method of not only reducing weight but also eliminating the stubborn lower-stomach fat. But why is it so?

First off, fasting optimizes the biological functions of your body. Fasting allows you to ease the load on your digestive system. The spare energy goes toward optimizing your physiological functions. For instance, improved digestion streamlines your bowel movement too. This efficacy in the physiological functions creates a compounding effect that leads to the shedding of dead weight, thus reducing an individual's weight and actually stabilizing it.

Another way in which fasting promotes weight loss is through cell autophagy. A dry fast is particularly what triggers cell autophagy. When the body uses up all its water, it now starts digesting the weak and damaged cells to provide water for the body cells that are in a much better state. Autophagy helps in eliminating dead and weak cells thereby making a person lighter.

Fasting plays a critical role in improving the metabolic health of an individual. With improved metabolism, the body can crunch more calories, and thus the individual's weight goes down.

Fasting improves insulin sensitivity. This helps the body to convert more sugars into energy. The body uses more calories, and as a result, there's a loss of weight.

In most obese people, the communication between their brain and ghrelin cells is warped, which makes them experience hunger all the time, even when they are full. Fasting helps remedy this problem, and obese people start receiving accurate signals when they are hungry.

Step-By-Step Process of Losing Weight through Fasting

- **Checkup**

First off, make sure that your body is in a condition that allows you to fast. Some of the people who are discouraged from the practice include pregnant women, nursing women, infants, sufferers of late-stage terminal illnesses, and those who are recovering from surgery.

- **Water**

Your body will respond to food deprivation by secreting acids and enzymes, and for that reason, always start your fast with consuming water. Regular water consumption will flush out the toxins and will also ease you from stomach pain.

- **Eating window**

Desist from food for at least 16 hours and then take a meal of your choice. The ideal eating window should be around eight hours. During this eight hour break, you are free to indulge. However, you must take care not to consume unhealthy foods. They will just neutralize your fasting efforts. Also, mind the portions. Simply because you have eight hours to feed doesn't mean you should fill up that period with food only.

- **Exercise**

Taking aerobic exercises, in particular, will have a dramatic effect on your weight loss. Aerobic exercises act like a calorie furnace. Also, exercises will increase the toxins in your body, and for that reason, keep yourself hydrated.

- **Breaking the fast**

At the end of your fast, never go right back into "heavy eating," but rather ease your way back by first consuming lighter foods. It'd be prudent of you to make fasting a part of your lifestyle. The key thing is to go with works for you. Most people seem to prefer intermittent fasting because it can fit in most people's lives. Prolonged fasting should be done sparingly as it carries the risk of developing complications.

Summary

Fasting has a positive impact on the rate of metabolism. When the metabolism rate is high, the energy output of the body goes up, and thus more calories are used up. This creates a caloric deficit and subsequent weight loss. Fasting promotes cell autophagy. Autophagy is the process where weak and damaged body cells are digested by the body. The elimination of weak body cells helps in weight reduction. High insulin resistance makes it hard for the body cells to absorb the sugars in the blood. But fasting reduces insulin resistance so that the body will use less insulin to convert sugars into energy. Before you go on a fast, you should get medical clearance. Some of the people who shouldn't get into a fast include the terminally ill, pregnant women, nursing women, and people who are recovering from surgery. It is important to take water throughout the fast to flush out toxins and mitigate the effect of stomach acids.

Chapter 11: Fasting for Type 2 Diabetes

What is Type 2 Diabetes?

Type 2 diabetes is a disease that damages the ability of the pancreas to produce sufficient insulin. Insulin is the hormone produced by the pancreas, and its main function is to regulate the conversion of glucose into energy. The body cells of people who have type 2 diabetes are insensitive to insulin, and as such, they experience difficulty in converting sugars into energy. This condition is known as insulin resistance. It is characterized by the production of higher amounts of insulin, but the body cannot absorb it.

As to the origin of type 2 diabetes, scientists have established that it is genetic. The disease is handed down to progeny. Another leading cause of type 2 diabetes is obesity. Overweight people are much more likely to develop insulin resistance. There's a link between childhood obesity and development of type 2 diabetes in adulthood.

Another contributing factor is a metabolic syndrome. High insulin resistance is a result of increased blood pressure and cholesterol. Excessive sugars produced by the liver may also be a trigger.

The symptoms of type 2 diabetes cover a wide range. They include thirst, frequent peeing, hazy vision, irritability, tiredness, and yeast infections.

The risk of developing type 2 diabetes can be greatly minimized by taking the following actions:

Losing weight. Weight loss improves insulin sensitivity, and thus the buildup of insulin in the blood is eliminated. Also, there's more conversion of sugars into energy.

Balanced diet. You should consume foods that are sources of minerals and vitamins. Increase your intake of fruits and vegetables. Minimize your consumption of sugars and red meat.

The Role of Insulin in the Body

The insulin hormone is produced by the pancreas. Its key role is to regulate blood sugar. Increased insulin resistance might lead to type 2 diabetes. Insulin plays the critical role of facilitating absorption of sugars into body cells. In this way, insulin helps to reduce the blood sugar level. Another important role of insulin is to modify the activity of enzymes. The enzymes are secreted by the body when there's food in the stomach. Insulin regulates the activity of enzymes.

Insulin helps the body recover quickly. When your body is recovering from an injury or illness, insulin plays a critical role in speeding up the healing process by transporting amino acids to cells.

Insulin promotes gut flora and thus improves gut health. This improves bowel movement. Insulin also improves the excretion of harmful substances like sodium.

Insulin promotes brain health. It improves brain clarity by providing the essential nutrients to the brain.

Insulin plays a key role in determining the metabolism rate of the body. In instances of high insulin sensitivity, the blood glucose is easily absorbed into the cells, making for a high metabolic rate. But in instances of low insulin sensitivity, the process of converting sugars into energy becomes hard, and, consequently, there is a low metabolic rate.

Insulin is very important in the optimal functioning of your body. Some of the factors that improve the production of the insulin hormone are having a balanced diet, improving your brain health, having quality sleep, exercising, and staying in a pollution-free environment.

How Diabetes Affects both Production and Usage of Insulin

Diabetes is a major lifestyle disease all over the world. A person who has diabetes either cannot produce sufficient insulin, or their body cells are insensitive to insulin. Diabetes is broadly classified into two types: type 1 and type 2.

People who suffer from type 1 diabetes produce little to no insulin. This slows down the rate of conversion of sugars into energy. A low level of insulin is mainly a result of the immune system attacking the pancreas and curtailing its ability to produce sufficient insulin. Also, low insulin levels might be a result of weakened and damaged body cells. Type 1 diabetes commonly affects young people. One of the corrective measures is to administer insulin through injections.

Symptoms of type 1 diabetes include dehydration, constant urge to urinate, hunger (even after eating), unexplained weight loss, blurry vision, exhaustion, and bad moods.

Type 2 diabetes is the most common form of diabetes. People who suffer from type 2 diabetes have a high insulin resistance. Their body cells are averse to insulin. Types 2 diabetes is treated by increasing insulin sensitivity.

Symptoms of type 2 diabetes include tiredness, never-ending thirst, constant urge to pee, irritability, weak immune, and shivering.

The pancreas is the organ that produces insulin. When we consume food, blood sugar rises. The pancreas releases insulin to facilitate the conversion of sugars into energy. But someone who suffers from diabetes either lacks sufficient insulin or their body cannot use the released insulin. This results in increased blood sugar levels. This scenario presents risks such as the development of heart disease and stroke.

How Blood Sugar Responds To Fasting

A carbohydrate metabolism test is crucial in determining how blood sugar responds to fasting. The test is conducted on diabetics. During a fast, the levels of plasma glucose go up. People with diabetes either cannot produce sufficient insulin, or their bodies are resistant to insulin. Non-diabetics, though, produce insulin that brings down the levels of glucose through absorption.

Diet greatly affects the blood sugar rate-of-increase. For instance, a big serving of food will trigger a high level of blood sugar, and sugar-laden foods like cake, bread, and fries will also increase the blood sugar level.

People with type 1 diabetes lack sufficient insulin because their immune system attacks the pancreas, while people with type 2 diabetes are insensitive to insulin. So in both cases, there is a high level of blood sugar.

The levels of blood glucose during fasting give us insight into how the cells respond to blood sugar. A high level of blood glucose is indicative of the body's ability to lower blood glucose, and the conclusion might be either high insulin resistance or insufficient insulin production. Prolonged fasting has the effect of minimizing blood glucose levels. The sugars in the blood get used up, albeit slowly.

There are two methods of testing the level of blood sugar: the traditional blood sugar test, and the glycosylated hemoglobin (HbAlc). The glycosylated hemoglobin test is for checking how blood glucose has been changing. The traditional method of checking blood sugar involves daily tests which may be conducted by the affected person.

Developing Your Fasting Regimen

There are some fasting regimens. All of them have their pros and cons. They are only as good as the person trying to follow them. During fasts, it is recommended to take water to flush out toxins and also to mitigate hunger. However, if you want to improve the success rate of your fast, you might consider dry fasts, where you don't consume any fluid.

You may perform a fast for as short a time as a couple of hours or as long as a full week (and maybe even more, depending on your stamina). However, if your goal is to lose weight, then shorter fasts are more effective. For instance, intermittent fasting is many times more fruitful than prolonged fasting, but ultimately, you get to choose what you feel will work for you.

Short fasts allow you to go through a cycle of fasting and eating windows. You start by creating a plan in which you detail your period of fasting and when your eating window opens. During the eating window, it is advisable to consume unprocessed foods and avoid sugar-laden foods. This will boost your insulin sensitivity.

Long fasts have their benefits too, but on the whole, they are much less rewarding than short fasts. The strain associated with long fasts make you susceptible to infections and might, in the worst case scenario, rewire your physiological functions.

Things to Incorporate to Make Fasting Safe for Diabetics

When a diabetic goes on a fast, their body secretes the glucagon hormone, which leads to a spike in the blood sugar level. Thus, a diabetic should start by informing themselves properly before they deprive themselves of food.

The first thing is to determine whether they are fit to fast. A diabetic person should seek medical clearance before they attempt fasting. A person with advanced diabetes will have a low blood sugar level. If they go on a fast, they risk falling into a coma. A medical professional offers the best counsel as to how to conduct the fast and for how long.

For type 1 diabetics, it is important to have a test kit to observe the fluctuation of blood sugar throughout the fast. This helps in tweaking the fast or deciding whether to call it off.

Another safety measure is to have a confidant know of their fasting. The psycho-social support offered by a confidant would keep them going. The confidant should be someone in their close proximity that can monitor their progress.

Diabetics should indulge in a balanced diet during their eating window. A balanced diet comprises of foods rich in minerals and vitamins. One common thing that fasting induces is cravings. Fast foods, for instance, are sugar-laden and they have no real nutritional value. Indulging in fast foods during eating windows only negates the effectiveness of the fast.

A diabetic should know when to quit and how to quit. If there is a massive fluctuation of blood glucose, or if a complication develops, then that's a hint to quit. Towards the end of the fast, a diabetic should consume light meals first, and then transition back to their normal eating patterns.

Role of Supplements

A supplement is a substance that enhances the food that a person eats. The common types of ingredients in supplements include vitamins, minerals, botanicals, amino acids, enzymes, organ tissues, and glandulars. The supplements are critical in optimizing nutritional value of food. The water-soluble ingredients of supplements are metabolized and eliminated from the body same day, while fat-soluble elements may be stored in the body for several days or even weeks. Supplements may be taken on either a daily basis or alternately—depending on the elements they provide to the body. One should always seek the guidance of a medical professional about the number of supplements to consume.

Supplements are not as critical during short fasts as they are in prolonged fasts. The body is a store of many nutritional elements, and fasting induces the body to tap into its reservoirs, but it is still important to take supplements to discourage nutrition deficiency. Fat-soluble vitamins need to be taken alongside fats to make for easy absorption. They include vitamin A, vitamin D, vitamin E, and vitamin K. They are kept in body cells too. Water-soluble vitamins are eliminated on the same day, especially if your body is well hydrated. Water-soluble vitamins include B3, B2, B1, and acids. If you have a poor diet, water-soluble vitamins are stable sources of nutrition.

The primary function of supplements is to improve the nutritional value of a person's diet by supplying vital elements that are not easily accessible. Taking supplements while on a fast helps mitigate the side effects of fasting such as headaches and cramps.

Types of Supplements that Stabilize Electrolytes

Sodium. The intake of Sodium is dependent upon your level of physical activity. Generally, if you engage in tougher physical exercises, you should take a high dose. Sodium is vital in eliminating cramps and various pains in the body.

Potassium. This supplement is vital for the optimal functioning of the heart. Potassium deficiency is normally accompanied by problems such as increased heartbeat and blood pressure. Potassium also helps in the flow of blood. A person with potassium deficiency is bound to experience exhaustion and constant lethargic feeling.

Magnesium. People who are lacking in this vital nutrient experience a range of problems like low energy, anxiety, insomnia, indigestion, muscle aches, poor heart health, and migraines. Magnesium supplements help your body absorb magnesium at a higher rate. Magnesium should be taken alongside food as opposed to plainly for maximum health benefit.

Zinc. This supplement is very crucial in improving the health of an individual. It regulates appetite, improves taste, promotes weight loss, minimizes hair loss, mitigates digestive problems, and cures chronic fatigue. Additionally, zinc improves nerve health and boosts testosterone. Zinc, too, should be consumed alongside other meals for maximum health benefits.

Calcium. This supplement helps in strengthening the musculoskeletal frame of an individual, heart health, and reduces the risk of developing ailments like cancer and diabetes. Calcium and magnesium should be taken at separate times to avoid stunted absorption rates.

Iodine. Iodine is crucial in improving thyroid health. The thyroid gland secretes hormones that play a vital role in the basal metabolic rate.

How to Keep Insulin Levels Low

This hormone produced by the pancreas facilitates the absorption of sugars into body cells. The insulin levels should be stable for optimum metabolism to take place. High levels of insulin might lead to serious complications like high blood pressure. Someone with a high blood glucose level needs to lower their blood sugar level, else they may suffer serious health complications. Here are some of the ways to keep insulin levels low.

Diet. Your diet will have a direct impact on your blood sugar levels. Sugary, fat-laden foods will raise your blood glucose through the roof. On the other hand, a low-carb diet will help keep your blood glucose levels down.

Portion. There is a direct correlation between the portion of your food and your blood sugar levels. A giant portion of your favorite dish will lead to a surge in blood glucose. On the other hand, a small portion will keep your blood sugar stable. Bearing this in mind, you should aim to take small portions of food, as they minimize the fluctuation of blood glucose levels.

Exercise regularly. You can bring the high blood sugar levels down through exercise. When you exercise, your body powers your activities with the glucose in your blood. So exercises—and in particular, aerobics—can lead to low blood glucose levels.

Drink water constantly. Staying hydrated is also important in keeping the blood sugar level down. Water will flush out toxins and help streamline your metabolism.

Avoid alcohol. Alcohol not only lowers your inhibitions and makes you indulge in unhealthy foods like fries and roast meat, but it is also calorie-packed. If you aim to minimize your blood sugar, restrict your alcohol intake or drop it altogether.

What Causes Insulin Resistance?

Insulin is produced by the pancreas, and its work is to facilitate absorption of glucose into body cells. Insulin resistance is a condition where body cells are insensitive to insulin. For that reason, the rate of conversion of sugars into energy is affected. What are some of the causes of this condition?

Obesity. Most obese people have a ton of toxic elements stashed in their body. The combination of high blood sugar levels and toxic elements promote cellular inflammation. These cells naturally become insulin resistant.

Inactivity. Insulin resistance is common in people who hardly ever move their limbs. They don't perform any physical activity, so their energy requirement (output) is minimal. This creates some sort of "cell apathy" and promotes insulin resistance.

Sleep apnea. This is a sleep disorder characterized by faulty breathing. People who suffer from sleep apnea snore loudly and also feel tired after a night's sleep. Studies have shown a link between sleep apnea and development of insulin resistance in body cells.

High blood pressure. High blood pressure or hypertension is a degenerative medical issue where the blood pressure in blood vessels is more than 140/90 mmHg. Hypertension makes the heart's task of pumping out blood more difficult and may contribute to complications such as atherosclerosis, stroke, and kidney disease. Studies have shown a correlation between people with high blood pressure and the development of insulin resistance.

Smoking. The habit of smoking can give you many health complications. One of them is the risk of cancer development. Additionally, smoking seems to promote insulin resistance.

How Insulin Resistance Affects the Body

Insulin resistance makes it hard for the body cells to absorb sugars, which leads to high blood glucose levels. Some of the causes of insulin resistance include obesity, poor diet, sleep disorders, and sedentary lifestyle.

The American Diabetes Association (ADA) has stated that there is a 70% chance for people with insulin resistance to develop type 2 diabetes if they don't change their habits.

Insulin resistance may trigger the development of acanthosis nigricans, a skin condition in which dark spots cover parts of the body, especially the neck region.

Insulin resistance enhances weight gain, because it slows down base metabolism, causing a surge of blood sugar levels. Insulin carries off the excess blood sugar into fat stores, and thus, the person gains weight.

Insulin resistance promotes high blood pressure. The elevated blood glucose levels cause the heart to have to struggle with pumping more blood, causing high blood pressure.

Insulin resistance causes constant thirst and hunger pangs. Insulin resistance promotes the miscommunication between brain receptors and body cells. Thus, the brain activates the hunger hormone and makes the person eternally hungry. If not corrected, this leads to overeating and eventually chronic obesity.

Insulin resistance weakens the body. Insulin resistance leads to low energy output. And for that reason, the body doesn't have a lot of energy to use up, which makes the person feel (and look) weak.

Insulin resistance makes you urinate frequently; the condition affects the efficiency of physiological functions, and one of the results is a constant need to urinate.

Insulin resistance makes the body more susceptible to attack by diseases.

The Role of Amylin

Amylin is a protein hormone. It is produced by the pancreas alongside insulin. Amylin helps in glycemic control by promoting the slow emptying of the gastric and giving feelings of satisfaction. Amylin discourages the upsurge of blood glucose levels.

Amylin is part of the endocrine system, and it plays a critical role in glycemic control. The hormone is secreted by the pancreas, and its main function is to slow down the rate of appearance of nutritional elements in the plasma. It complements insulin.

Amylin and Insulin are secreted in a ratio of 1:100. Amylin delays gastric emptying and decreases the concentration of glucose in the plasma, whereas insulin facilitates absorption of sugars into cells. Diabetic people lack this hormone.

The amylin hormone can coalesce and create amyloid fibers, which may help in destroying diabetes. Amylin is secreted when there is the stimulus of nutrition in the blood. Unlike insulin, it is not purged in the liver but by renal metabolism.

Recent studies have shown the effect of amylin on the metabolism of glucose. In rats, amylin promoted insulin resistance.

Amylin slows down the food movement through the gut. As the food stays longer in the stomach, the rate of conversion of these foods to sugars will be slower.

Amylin also prevents the secretion of glucagon. Glucagon causes a surge in blood sugar level. Amylin prevents the inappropriate secretion of glucagon, which might cause a post-meal spike in blood sugar.

Amylin enhances the feeling of satiety. By reducing appetite, amylin ensures low blood glucose levels.

How Amylin Deficiency Affects Your Body

Amylin regulates the concentration of glucose in the blood by preventing the secretion of glucagon and slowing down the movement of food along the gut. People who suffer from diabetes have an amylin deficiency that causes excessive amounts of glucose to flow into the blood.

Increased insulin. A deficiency in amylin causes an extreme surge in blood glucose levels. To mitigate this spike, the pancreas secretes more insulin to help in the absorption of sugars into body cells. Increased levels of insulin in the blood might lead to complications.

Insulin resistance. Amylin deficiency eventually leads to high blood glucose levels. This might cause insulin resistance in body cells and, in worst case scenarios, it might trigger the immune system to attack the pancreas. High insulin levels in the blood might trigger memory loss and might even induce a coma.

Diabetes. Amylin deficiency leads to the overproduction of insulin, which, in the long run, impairs the pancreas. When the normal working of the pancreas is damaged, diabetes may develop.

Weight gain. Amylin deficiency promotes insulin resistance. When body cells become insensitive to insulin, there is less sugar converted into energy. So, the blood glucose level remains high. Insulin is responsible for carrying off these sugars to be stored as fats. Instead of these sugars being used as energy, they end up being stored as fat in the cells, which is the start of weight gain.

Headache. Thanks to insulin resistance, the body cells lack a reliable source of energy, which causes the body to switch to burning fats as an alternative energy source. One of the side effects of this process is normally headache and nausea.

The Insulin Resistance Diet

Insulin resistance causes slower absorption of sugars into body cells. This condition is rampant in obese people and diabetics. It is projected that the number of diabetics in the next 20 years will be over 320 million. This indicates a very worrying trend of diabetes. One of the things we can do to fight against diabetes is to improve our diet. Studies have shown that weight loss is a very effective means of minimizing insulin resistance. Here are the components of an insulin resistant diet:

Low carbs. Food high in carbs are responsible for blood sugar spikes. High levels of blood glucose promote insulin resistance. To ensure a stable blood glucose level, you should stick to low-carb foods.

Avoid sugary drinks. The American Diabetes Association advises against consumption of sugary drinks. These drinks with high sugar content include fruit juice, corn syrup, and other concentrates. Sugary drinks have a high sugar content, and they spike blood sugar levels. So, it'd be prudent to stay away from sugary drinks.

More fiber. Fiber is important in reducing the blood glucose levels. It improves the digestive health and improves blood circulation.

Healthy fats. Monounsaturated fats are very critical in improving heart health and regulating insulin levels.

Protein. Studies show that dietary protein is beneficial for people who suffer from diabetes. Regular consumption of protein is important for muscle growth and bone mass.

Size. Instead of taking large servings of a meal, opt for smaller portions of food, so that your post-meal blood glucose levels may be stable.

The Best Food for Diabetics

Diabetics don't have the luxury of eating any food they might want. For instance, sugar-laden foods and high-fat foods would spike their blood sugar levels and worsen the condition. They should instead stick to foods that are sources of minerals and vitamins. Foods like:

Fish. Fish is an important source of omega-3 fatty acids. These fatty acids are especially great for people with heart health complications and those who are at risk of stroke. Omega three fatty acids also protect your blood vessels, as well as reduce inflammation. Studies show that people who consume fish on the regular have better heart health than those who don't.

Greens. They are very nutritious and have low calories. Leafy greens like kale and spinach are excellent sources of minerals and vitamins. Leafy greens reduce inflammation markers, as well improve blood pressure. They are also high in antioxidants.

Eggs. The good old egg has been abused at the hands of intellectual conmen who have long said, albeit incorrectly, that eggs are bad. Eggs are excellent for reducing heart disease complications and also decreasing inflammation markers. Regular consumption of eggs improves cholesterol and blood glucose levels.

Chia seeds. They are high in fiber, and this fiber is critical in lowering blood glucose levels as well as in slowing down the rate of movement of food along the gut.

Nuts. Nuts are both tasty and healthy. They are great sources of fiber and are low in carbs. Regular consumption improves heart health and reduces inflammation and improves blood circulation.

Summary

Type 2 diabetes is a degenerative disease that impairs the ability of the pancreas to produce insulin. The hormone insulin is produced by the pancreas, and its main function is to regulate the conversion of glucose to energy. The risk of developing diabetes can be greatly minimized by taking the two steps: losing weight and having a balanced diet. The number of people with diabetes is at an all-time high, and people in both developed and poor countries are battling the disease. Symptoms of type 2 diabetes include tiredness, never-ending thirst, the constant urge to pee, irritability, weak immune system, and shivering. A carbohydrate metabolism test determines how blood sugar reacts to fasting. During a fast, blood sugar levels go up. Supplements are necessary for supplying important nutrients that may not be in the diet. The intake of supplements should be daily for optimum results. The important supplements include sodium, potassium, magnesium, zinc, calcium, and iodine. These are some of the measures to take to keep insulin levels low: have a strict diet, consume small portions, exercise regularly, and drink water constantly.

Chapter 12: Fasting For Heart Health

How Fasting Improves Your Heart's Health

Numerous studies have shown that fasting has a positive impact on heart health. Many people who have gone on a fast have reported feeling energetic and livelier afterward, which could be attributed to improved blood flow and general heart health. However, you need to fast consistently to achieve results.

Improves your heartbeat. When you go on a fast, your body is free from the digestion load, and so it channels that energy into optimizing your physiological functions. Your heart stands to gain from the optimized body functions, especially improving your heartbeat.

Improves blood pressure. Studies show that fasting has a positive impact on blood pressure. The rate of blood pressure is affected by factors like weight gain and obesity. But since fasting helps in weight loss, it has the extended advantage of lowering blood pressure, which improves the overall heart health.

Reduces cholesterol. Regularly fasting helps in lowering bad cholesterol. Also, controlled fasting increases the base metabolic rate.

Improved blood vessel health. Fasting is critical in improving the health of blood vessels. When blood vessels are subjected to high blood pressure, they slowly start to wear out, and might eventually burst up— which could be fatal, especially in the case of arteries. But fasting helps reduce blood pressure and bad cholesterol. The result is improved blood flow and overall heart health.

Autophagy. Regular dry fasts trigger the body to digest its weak and damaged cells in a process known as autophagy. Cell autophagy is very crucial because it helps eliminate old and damaged cells and creates room for new cells. With a new batch of cells to work with, the heart health is given a tremendous boost.

Summary

Fasting has been shown to improve the health of the heart. When you are fasting, your body reserves energy that would have gone into digestion for purposes of improving the heart health. It can execute its physiological functions much better. Fasting has also been shown to improve blood pressure. Fasting helps reduce obesity and reduces weight gain. This causes massive improvement in blood pressure. Fasting also plays a critical role in reducing cholesterol. Bad cholesterol increases the rate of developing heart disease. Also, controlled fasting increases the base metabolic rate. Fasting also improves the health of blood vessels. High blood pressure might cause blood vessels to wear out slowly, but fasting has a restorative effect on the blood vessels. Fasting also allows the body to digest its weak cells and make room for new and powerful body cells.

Chapter 13: The General Results of Fasting

Positive Effects of Fasting

You will get varied results depending on your preferred method of fasting, whether it's intermittent fasting, alternate-day, or prolonged fasting. These are some of the positive effects of fasting:

Weight loss. Fasting is an efficient way of losing weight. A study in 2015 showed that alternate fasting for a week resulted in weight loss of up to seven percent. When your body uses up the glucose in your blood, it now turns to the fat reserves to power its bodily functions. This helps in achieving weight loss.

Release of the human growth hormone. The human growth hormone promotes the growth of muscles and reduces obesity. Fasting triggers the secretion of the human growth hormone. This hormone is very crucial in building your body cells.

Improves insulin sensitivity. Low insulin sensitivity restricts the absorption of sugars into body cells. This might lead to complications such as chronic weight gain. Fasting leads to high insulin sensitivity that helps in absorption of sugars into body cells.

Normalizes ghrelin levels. Ghrelin is the hunger hormone which sends out hunger signals. Most obese people have abnormal ghrelin hormone levels that keep them in a perpetual state of hunger. Fasting, however, remedies this situation by normalizing ghrelin hormone levels, and thus you can receive accurate signals about hunger.

Lowers triglyceride levels. Depriving yourself of food for a set period of time has the effect of lowering bad cholesterol, and in the process, triglycerides are reduced.

Slows down aging. Many studies have shown the link between fasting and increased longevity in animals. Fasting allows the body to cleanse itself, promotes cell autophagy, and in the long run, lengthens lifespan.

Negative Effects of Fasting

As much as fasting is a practice with many benefits, admittedly there is a dark side too. These are some of the negative effects of fasting:

Strained body. A prolonged fast might put a big deal of a strain on your body. This may alter—albeit slightly—the normal processes of your body. A prolonged fast might slow down the effectiveness of your body as the body adapts to survive on too little energy.

Headaches. Headaches are common during fasts, especially at the start. The headache is normally a response of the brain to diminished blood glucose levels that force the body to switch to burning fats as a source of energy.

Low blood pressure. Fasting is a major cause of low blood pressure. Low blood pressure slows down the conversion of sugars into energy. This may lead to complications such as temporary blindness and, in extreme cases, can induce a coma.

Eating disorders. For someone who's too eager, it is easy to abuse fasting and turn it into an eating disorder. The main aim of fasting is to improve health, but starving yourself and having an eating disorder is anything but healthy. Some of the eating disorders that people who fast are at risk of developing include anorexia and bulimia.

Cravings. The hunger triggered by fasting might cause us to overcompensate. We may develop cravings for fast foods and other unhealthy foods. During our eating window, we may find ourselves consuming a lot of unhealthy foods, under the delusion that the fast will override that.

Summary

Weight loss is one of the main benefits of fasting. When you fast, your blood glucose is diminished, and this forces your body to turn to fats as an alternative source of energy. Fasting also promotes the production of the human growth hormone. This is the hormone responsible for muscle growth. Fasting also improves insulin sensitivity. Low insulin sensitivity impairs the body's ability to convert sugars into energy. Fasting also leads to high insulin sensitivity that helps in the absorption of sugars into body cells. Fasting also helps normalize ghrelin levels. The ghrelin hormone is known as the hunger hormone. Most obese people have abnormally high ghrelin levels that give incorrect hunger signals and make the obese person perpetually hungry. Fasting helps in correcting this problem, and the obese person starts to receive accurate signals. The negative effects of fasting include straining the body, headaches, low blood pressure, and eating disorders.

Part 4: Important Factors that Improve the Quality of Fasting

Chapter 14: Nutrition

What Constitutes Good Nutrition?

Good nutrition implies a diet that contains all the required and important nutrients in appropriate proportions. When you fail to observe good nutrition, you risk developing complications from certain nutrient deficiencies. A good nutrition shouldn't be a one-off thing, but it should be a part of your lifestyle.

A great nutrition minimizes the risk of developing health complications such as diabetes, heart disease, and chronic weight gain. Here are the most important constituents of great nutrition:

- **Protein**

This nutrient is very important for muscle health, skin health, and hair. Also, it assists in the bodily reactions. Amino acids are essential for human growth and protein is stacked with amino acids. The best sources of protein include fish, eggs, and lentils.

- **Carbohydrates**

Carbohydrates are the main sources of energy for the body. They provide sugars that are converted into energy. There are two classes of carbohydrates: simple and complex. Simple carbohydrates are digested easily, and complex carbohydrates take time. Fruits and grains are some of the main sources of simple carbohydrates whereas beans and vegetables are sources of complex carbohydrates. For proper digestion, dietary fiber (carbohydrate) is needed. Men need a daily intake of 30 grams of fiber and women need 24 grams. Important sources of dietary fiber include legumes and whole grains.

- **Fats**

Fats play an essential role in health improvement. Both monounsaturated and polyunsaturated fats are healthy. Sources of monounsaturated fats include avocados and nuts. As for polyunsaturated fats, seafood is a major source. Unhealthy fats include trans fats and saturated fats, mostly found in junk food.

- **Vitamins**

Vitamins A, B, C, D, E, and K are necessary for the body's optimal functioning. A deficiency in the important vitamins can lead to serious health complications and weakened immune system.

- **Minerals**

Calcium, iron, zinc, and iodine are some of the essential minerals. They are found in a variety of foods including vegetables, grains, and meats.

- **Water**

Most of the human body is composed of water. It is a very essential nutrient for the proper functioning of the body.

Why Good Nutrition Is Important
The main reason why people ensure that they have a good nutrition is to improve their health. A good nutrition is essentially about consuming foods that are rich in vitamins, minerals, and fats. So, here are some of the

reasons why good nutrition is vital.

Reduces risk of cancer. Good nutrition plays a vital role in optimizing your health. If you consume healthy food, you drastically reduce your chances of getting cancer, as many cancers are a result of bad lifestyle choices.

Reduces risk of developing high blood pressure. High blood pressure causes a strain on the heart. It also leads to the wearing and tearing of the blood vessels. Having good nutrition normalizes your blood pressure and thus improves your heart health.

Lowers cholesterol. Bad cholesterol leads to serious complications like heart disease. When you observe good nutrition that involves fruits and essential vitamins, the bad cholesterol is eliminated, thus improving the functioning of your body.

Increased energy. Bad food choices have a draining effect. However, nutritious foods replenish the body cells with vital nutrients, and thus the body is active. A nutritious diet is a key to improving productivity.

Improved immunity. Diseases are always looking for new victims. People who have a poor diet are bound to have a weak immune system. The weak immune system won't sufficiently protect them against attacks. On the other hand, people who consume a nutritious diet tend to have a strong immune system. This improved immunity keeps diseases at bay.

The Advantages of a High-Fat Diet

Many studies have shown that a low-carb, high-fat diet has many health benefits, including weight management, and reduced risk of diabetes, cancer, and Alzheimer's. A high-fat diet is characterized by low carbohydrate intake and high intake of fat. The low carbohydrate intake puts the body into ketosis, a condition that optimizes burning of fat and helps convert fat into ketone bodies that act as an energy source of the brain. These are some of the advantages of a high-fat diet:

Stronger immune system. Saturated fats are an ally of the immune system. They help fight off microbes, viruses, and fungi. Fats help in the fight against diseases. A great source of saturated fats includes butter and coconut.

Improves skin health and eyesight. When someone is lacking in fatty acids, they are likely to develop dry skin and eyes. Fatty acids help in improving skin elasticity and strengthening eyesight.

Lowers risk of heart disease. Saturated fats trigger production of good cholesterol, which is key in reducing the risk of heart disease. Saturated fats also help fight inflammation. A good source of saturated fats includes eggs and coconut oil.

Strong bones. Healthy fats improve the density of bones and thus minimize the risk of bone diseases. Fats promote healthy calcium metabolism. Fatty acids, too, play a critical role in minimizing the risk of bone complications such as osteoporosis.

Improves reproductive health. Fats play a critical role in the production of hormones that improve fertility in both men and women. A high-fat diet improves reproductive health and, in particular, the production of testosterone and estrogen.

Weight loss. A high-fat diet promotes high metabolism and, as a result, the body can crunch more calories, leading to weight loss.

Improved muscle gain. A high-fat diet promotes muscle gain. This is achieved through hormone production and speeding up cell recovery after strenuous exercise.

Role of Ketone Bodies

The three ketone bodies produced by the liver include acetoacetate, beta-hydroxybutyrate, and acetone. Ketone bodies are water-soluble, and it takes a blood or urine test to determine their levels.

Ketone bodies are oxidized in the mitochondria to provide energy. The heart uses fatty acids as fuel in normal circumstances, but during ketogenesis, it switches to ketone bodies. When the blood glucose levels are high, the body stores the excesses as fat. When you go for an extended period of time without eating, the blood glucose levels diminish. This triggers the body to convert fat into usable energy. Most body cells can utilize fatty acids, except the brain. The liver thus converts fats into ketone bodies and releases them into the blood to supply energy to the brain. When ketone bodies start to build up in the blood, problems might arise. An increase in the levels of acetone can induce acidosis, a condition where blood pH is lowered. Acidosis has a negative impact on most of the body cells, and in worst cases, it leads to death. With that in mind, it is prudent to replenish your body with carbohydrates as soon as ketosis kicks off. A person with type 1 diabetes is more susceptible to high levels of ketone bodies. For instance, when they fail to take an insulin shot, they will experience hypoglycemia. The combination of low blood glucose level and high glucagon level will cause the liver to produce ketone bodies at an alarming rate which might cause complications.

Benefits of the Ketogenic Diet

Here are some of the benefits associated with ketone bodies:

Treating Alzheimer's. Alzheimer's behaves in a way similar to diabetes. Essentially, it is the brain resisting insulin. Due to insulin resistance, the brain only gets minimal energy, which might cause the death of brain cells. However, ketone bodies are an alternative source of energy that the brain can utilize. Ketone bodies have been shown to prevent a buildup of compounds that enhance the development of Alzheimer.

Normalizes insulin production. Ketone bodies are only produced when blood glucose is low. For this reason, the pancreas stops pumping more insulin to aid in the absorption of sugars because the body has already switched into ketogenesis.

Regulates metabolism. Ketone bodies regulate metabolism through their effects on mitochondria. The mitochondria are the cells' power plants, and they respond better to energy from fats rather than glucose. In this sense, ketone bodies improve the functioning of the mitochondria.

Lowers hunger. When the body is utilizing ketone bodies, it seems that there's less of an urge to consume food. Ketogenesis regulates the hunger hormone. When a person is consuming fast foods, there is no end to the urge to take another serving. Eventually, this leads to weight gain.

Increases good cholesterol. The good cholesterol improves blood flow and the condition of your heart. Ketogenesis helps in the production of the good cholesterol and thus helps in improving heart health.

Improves brain health. Ketone bodies are especially effective as a source of energy for the brain. Many people who have practiced the ketone diet say that it improves their mental clarity and focus.

The Importance of a Well-Balanced Diet

When we talk about a balanced diet, we refer to a variety of foods that supply us with important nutrients such as protein, carbohydrates, healthy fats, vitamins, and minerals. So, what is the importance of a well-balanced diet?

Strengthens immune system. When you consume a diet that's rich in nutrients, your immune system will become stronger. This places your body in a far better place to fight disease vectors that might have otherwise overwhelmed your body's defense system.

Weight loss. In the past, obesity was a problem in only developed nations. Not anymore. Nowadays even poor people are struggling with obesity. This is partially due to fast foods being cheaper and more convenient. As you can imagine, obesity has become a crisis the world over. The open secret is that obesity can be mitigated through a balanced diet. A diet rich in nutritious elements will nourish your body and also regulate your appetite so that you don't fall into the temptation of eating unhealthy foods.

Mental health. People who observe a balanced diet are less likely to fall into bad moods and depression. The nutritious elements stabilize their emotions and enable them to be more resistant to the autosuggestions of their mind.

Skin health. Dry skin is often the result of a bad diet. When you have a balanced diet, your skin and hair are nourished, and it gives you a glow. Foods rich in vitamins and collagen improve skin elasticity.

Promotes growth. A balanced diet helps kids have a well-formed body as they transition into adults and it helps adults maintain a well-figured body.

Summary

A good nutrition is a diet that contains all the important nutrients in appropriate portions. You risk developing complications if you fail to follow a good nutrition. The risk of developing health complications is greatly minimized by a great nutrition. Protein is one of the most important elements of a good nutrition. It is important for muscle health, skin health and development of hair. Protein also plays a role in bodily reactions. Carbohydrates are the major source of energy. They provide glucose that the body cells use to power activities of the body. Fats also play an important role in improving health. Monounsaturated fats and polyunsaturated fats are especially healthy. Vitamins are necessary for the body to function optimally. Minerals and water are important too. People ensure that they have good nutrition to improve their health. They achieve this by consuming foods that are rich in nutritious elements. A high-fat diet promotes strong immunity, better eyesight, a lower risk of heart disease, and stronger bones.

Chapter 15: Exercise

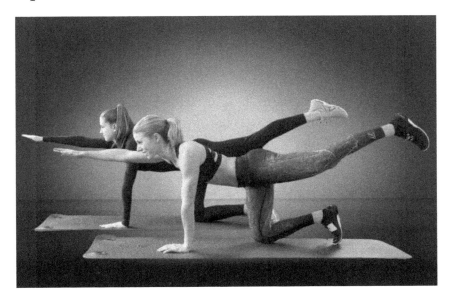

Pros of Exercising While Fasting

For the longest time, it was considered unhealthy to exercise while on a fast, but new evidence has shown that it is perfectly healthy to exercise even while you are fasting.

When you fast for health purposes, it shows that you are committed to improving your health and managing your weight. One of the ways you could get better results is by turning to physical exercise. A combination of intermittent fasting and physical exercise will burn up calories and help you reach your health goals in the shortest time possible.

The time of day that you exercise seems to affect the outcome. For instance, exercising in the morning right after you wake up promotes more weight loss than exercising at night. For intermittent fasting to be effective, you need to abstain from food for at least 16 hours.

When you exercise while on a fast, you speed up weight loss and optimize your health because of increased oxidation that promotes the growth of muscle cells.

It enriches your blood. Exercising has a positive effect on your breathing system and lung capacity. This helps in increasing the oxygen levels in your blood.

Exercising also improves heart health. Aerobic exercises, in particular, improve blood circulation and develop the stamina of the heart. Now, the blood pressure stabilizes and nutrients can spread to the whole body.

Exercising while on a fast improves your body's adaptability. It is never a good idea to idle around while on a fast, as it will trigger cravings. However, when you engage in physical activity, your body starts to adapt. It helps you create more stamina to endure your fast.

Best Exercises to Do

Exercising while fasting increases the rate of calorie burning. As a result, more weight is lost, and health is optimized in much less time. Here are the best exercises to perform while on a fast:

- **Aerobic exercise**

Aerobic exercise increases your heartbeat and breathing cycle. Aerobic exercise also improves lung capacity and heart health. Some of the benefits of aerobic exercise include improved mental health, minimized inflammation, lowered blood pressure, lowered blood sugar, and a minimized risk of heart disease, stroke, type 2 diabetes, and cancer. Aerobic exercises tend to be intense and easy to perform. Some examples of aerobic exercises include dancing, speed-walking, jogging, and cycling.

- **Strength training**

Strength training is important for muscle gain. People who perform strength training have more energy and keep their bodies at peak performance. Strength training improves your mental health, decreases blood sugar levels, enhances weight management, corrects posture, increases balance, and relieves pain in the back and joints. Strength training may be performed either in the gym or at home. Professional guidance depends on the exact exercise and equipment required. Strength training mostly takes the form of exercises such as pull-ups, push-ups, sit-ups, squats, and lunges. It is recommended to take breaks from strength training to allow muscle growth.

- **Stretching**

Stretching exercises are vital in improving the flexibility of a person. The exercises are designed to improve the strength and flexibility of tendons. Stretching exercises also improve the aesthetic quality of muscles. They also improve the circulation of blood and promote nourishment of all body cells.

- **Balance exercises**

Balance exercises promote agility. The exercises are designed to make your joints flexible. Balance exercises lead to improved focus and motor skills. The exercises include squats, sit-ups, and leg lifts.

Summary

Contrary to what people thought for the longest time, it is healthy to exercise while on a fast. A combination of exercise and fasting is a resource-intensive activity that makes your body burn more calories. Studies show that exercising in the morning has a far better outcome than exercising at night before bed. When you exercise while fasting, oxidation in cells promotes the growth of muscles. Exercising while on a fast also enriches your blood. The improved breathing cycle and lung capacity help in increasing the level of oxygen in the blood. Exercising is vital in improving heart health and blood circulation. It is never a good idea to stay idle while you are on a fast. Your hunger will be magnified, and it might cause to break the fast. Some of the best exercises to do for maximum weight loss and health improvement include aerobic exercises, strength training, stretching and balance exercises.

Chapter 16: Having a Partner to Keep You in Check

Role of a Partner

Depriving yourself of food is by no means easy. If you have no experience, the temptation to slide back is real. In some instances, fasting might make you lapse into a worse state than before. This is especially after a small duration of fasting where the hunger is extreme, and then you are tempted into eating unhealthy foods, trapping you into eating them.

Having a partner to keep you in check is a good step, and if they are into fasting themselves, that's even better. Ideally, your partner should be someone that "understands" you. He or she will make fasting less taxing. They will be there to see your progress and offer constructive criticism when needed. As your fasting progresses, they will help you adjust accordingly or make tweaks, to go through the fast in the safest manner possible.

Your partner will hold you accountable for your fasting journey. Attaining health goals is no easy task. It takes dedication, discipline, and consistency. It's exactly why you need a partner to hold you accountable when you stray or when you fall back on your goals. A responsible partner will be interested in your gains (i.e., asking questions about your weight loss so far and wanting to know what your diet is like).

A partner is also important because you have someone to talk to about your journey. They can offer you psychosocial support in your moments of vulnerability. It makes a world of difference. And you will stick to your goals knowing that someone cares.

Traits to Look for in a Partner

Not everyone may qualify to be a partner to someone who's fasting. The first thing to look out for is their opinion on the subject of fasting. Some people seem to think that fasting is a bad practice and a waste of time. Clearly, you wouldn't want such a person as your partner.

- **Patience**

Your partner should demonstrate patience. You cannot rush things while fasting. Sometimes, the results might take time, and in such situations, the last thing you want is someone on your neck, probably trashing your methods.

- **Observation skills**

A great partner must be a good observer. Their job is to spot loopholes that need to be closed, to assess situations, and to weigh overall progress. They need strong observation skills that will make them suitable for their positions. Also, remember that it is sometimes critical to call off a fast. Maybe you will be hard on yourself even when you are falling apart. An observant partner should notice the change and suggest that you stop.

- **Communication skills**

They should have good communication skills. What good is it to know something and not express it in a timely and appropriate fashion? A great partner should be very communicative and should express him/herself in an elaborate manner.

- **Knowledgeable**

A good partner should be knowledgeable. They should have a working knowledge of the whole subject of fasting. During every step of the fast, they should have a mental picture of what's coming. This will strengthen your bond and together you can meet any challenge.

- **Respect**

They should be able to respect you, your methods, and also have self-respect. This creates an enabling environment.

Should You Join A Support Group?

When your brain floods you with hunger hormones during a fast, the temptation to quit is real. One of the methods to minimize your chances of quitting is to join a support group. This is ideally a group of people who have similar fasting pursuits as you. Now you have a family to keep you in check and boost your confidence.

A support network will allow you to cope and express your feelings and get connected with like-minded people. In times of vulnerability, others will come to your help. As other members share their experiences, you learn that you are not alone, and you even broaden your perspective and wisdom.

Support networks include people who are at various stages toward the common goal you all have. In times of conflict, you have ready help, and if you are at an advanced stage yourself, then you should offer help to those in need of it too. Support networks have non-judgmental environments and therapeutic effects.

The best support groups are those that foster frequent get-togethers. Ideally, the members should come from the same society, but that doesn't mean other kinds of support groups are necessary. For instance, you could join an online support network and be free to commune with your family at your convenience. Online support groups seem to be a thing nowadays. People from around the world with common goals are coming together to form support networks.

The most important thing when you join a support group is to become a giver rather than a taker. Or both. When everyone is interested in giving, you have a resourceful group of like-minded people.

Summary

People who are overwhelmed by the idea of staying without food should consider getting a partner. Your partner should help you cultivate a strong sense of discipline and stick to your routine. Ideally, your partner should be someone who understands you. He or she will help you get through fasting. A supportive partner is there to check your progress and offer constructive criticism when the occasion calls for it. He or she should be someone that you can open up to and express your fears and concerns. With the right partner, your fasting journey will be smooth and enjoyable. Your partner should be patient, observant, communicative, respectful, and knowledgeable. Joining a support group will help you come together with other like-minded people for a common goal. You are guaranteed of ready help and psychosocial support. The best support group to join should comprise of people from your local area, but it doesn't rule out joining even online support groups and communing with people from different parts of the world.

Chapter 17: Motivation

How to Stay Motivated Throughout Your Fast

Get a partner. If you go it alone, you are much more likely to forgive yourself and tweak the fast to suit you. For that reason, let there be a person to whom you are accountable. This person should put you in check and ensure that you follow the rules. Offer constructive criticism, and suggestions. A partner will help you stick to your routine. The ideal partner should be patient, empathetic, a good communicator, and knowledgeable about fasting. Let them share in your accomplishments as much as they have shared in your trials and struggle.

Seek knowledge. Being informed makes all the difference. You will know every possible outcome. You are aware of all the side effects of fasting and how to persist through the unpleasant experience instead of just quitting. Knowledge will help you optimize your fast and make you reap more benefits than anyone who had just deprived themselves of food. Being knowledgeable is important also in the sense that you are more aware of when to stop.

Set goals. Don't get into fasting with mental blindness. Instead, make an effort to set milestones. When you achieve a goal—for instance, when you hit your target weight—celebrate and then go back to reducing weight. Your brain responds to victory by making you feel confident. Now, you will have more confidence in your capacity to withstand hunger.

Develop positivity. A positive attitude makes all the difference. Keep reading about successful people who have achieved what you are looking for. Lockout all the negative energies that would derail you.

Record your progress. It is easy to underestimate yourself. As long as you keep going, the achievements will always be there. It's just a matter of recognizing them and celebrating.

How to Make Fasting Your Lifestyle

There are different approaches to fasting. You may fast every other day, once a week, or even a couple of times every month. In each instance, there are benefits.

But if you'd like to reap great benefits out of fasting, you should purposefully make it a daily ritual. Many people in the world today fast on a daily basis and have reported an increased quality of life.

The most common and most rewarding method is the 16:8 intermittent fasting. In this method, you fast for 16 hours in a day and then eat during the other 8 hours to complete the cycle.

Ideally, when you wake up, you should take a drink of water or black coffee and either exercise or just go on about your work. At around noon, your eating window opens, and you're free to have your meals up until 8 pm when the eating window closes.

During this eight-hour eating window, it is common to be tempted to overeat or indulge in unhealthy foods, thinking that the coming fast will "take care of that." Well, you must be careful not to fall into this temptation, or else your gains will be negated. Consume healthy and nutritious foods during the eating window and adhere to your 16-hour fast. The weight loss starts occurring in as short a span as a few days.

If you incorporate intermittent fasting into your lifestyle, the weight loss keeps going until you hit a stable weight where it plateaus. When fasting is your lifestyle, it makes your health improvement and weight loss permanent.

Summary

You need to take a few measures to stay motivated throughout the fast. One of the measures is to get a partner. A partner should hold you accountable and keep you in check so that you don't stray from the fasting routine. The ideal partner should be patient, empathetic, and a good communicator. Another way of motivating yourself is through seeking knowledge. As a knowledgeable person, you will be aware of all the responses that your body will give off. Knowledge will also help you optimize your fast and get the best possible results. Other ways to stay motivated throughout the fast include setting goals, developing positivity and recording your progress. If you make fasting part of your lifestyle, you stand to reap more benefits. The most common and most efficient fasting method is the 16:8, where you fast for 16 hours and then have an eating window of 8 hours.

Chapter 18: Foods for the Fast

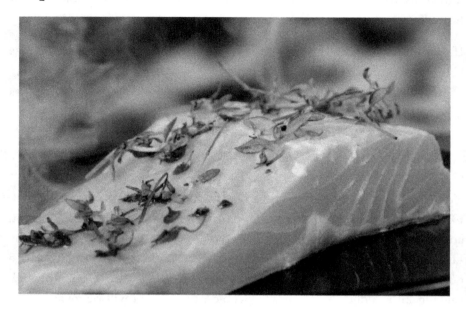

How Food Controls the Rate of the Success of Fasting

Depriving yourself of food is no easy task. Your body will tune up the hunger, and you will have to suppress the urge to feed. Not easy.

When you consume food, it is digested and released into the bloodstream as sugars. The pancreas secretes the hormone insulin to help in absorption of these sugars into body cells. When you stay for long without eating, there is no more food getting digested, and thus no more sugars getting released into the blood. The body soon runs out of the existing sugars and meets a crisis. The body is forced to switch to fats to provide energy for various physiological functions.

The foods that you eat have a massive impact on the efficacy of the fast. If you take light meals or small portions of food during the eating window, you will experience a higher degree of hunger during the fast. On the other side, if you consume large amounts of food during your eating window, your hunger will not be as intense.

One of the tricks to reducing hunger during the fast is to consume foods that are high in dietary fiber. Such foods make you full for a long time and will thus minimize the unpleasant feeling triggered by hunger.

Consuming healthy foods during your eating window is important. Some people fall into the temptation of eating unhealthy foods or even eating too much, and the effect is negative.

Intermittent fasting is favored by many people because it doesn't restrict consumption of foods, unlike fad diets that insist on vegan meals or raw food.

The Worst Foods to Take During Fasting

If you want to speed up your weight loss and avoid lifestyle diseases, these are some of the foods to cut back on, or maybe stay away from:

Sugary drinks. The high dose of fructose in sugary drinks will cause an extreme surge of blood sugar levels. High amounts of this kind of sugar promote insulin resistance and liver disease. High levels of insulin resistance have a negative impact on the absorption of sugars into body cells. This creates the perfect recipe for the development of heart disease and diabetes.

Junk food. They might taste heavenly, but the ingredients of most junk foods come from hell. Junk foods have almost zero nutritional value. Fries are prepared using hydrogenated oil that contains trans fats. Studies have been made on trans fats, and the conclusion is that continued consumption of trans fats leads to heart complications and cancer.

Processed food. Most processed foods have a long shelf life thanks to a host of nasty chemicals poured into them. The processed foods are made durable to gain a commercial edge over organic products with a limited shelf life. Most processed foods are high in sugars, sodium, and have low fiber content and nutrients.

White bread and cakes. Baked goods tend to affect people with celiac disease, most especially. But more than that, most of these baked goods are stashed with processed ingredients—sugars and fats—and they are low on fiber. Most baked goods trigger abnormal surges in blood sugar levels and increase the risk of heart disease.

Alcohol. Studies show that alcohol induces inflammation on the liver. Excessive alcohol consumption will eliminate all the successes of your fast and promote weight gain and even development of diabetes.

Seed oils. Studies show that these oils are unnatural. They contain harmful fatty acids that increase the risk of developing heart complications.

The Best Foods to Take During Fasting

These are some of the best foods to indulge in while you fast to reach your important health goals:

Nuts. Nuts are rich in nutritional value. Almonds, Brazil nuts, lentils, oatmeal, etc. have properties that help in the production of good cholesterol. Good cholesterol promotes heart health. Nuts are excellent sources of vitamins and minerals. Oatmeal, in particular, is essential in normalizing blood glucose levels.

Fruits and greens. They are important sources of essential nutrients that improve both gut health and brain health. Broccoli is rich in phytonutrients that reduce the risk of heart complications and cancers. Apples contain antioxidants that eliminate harmful radicals. Kale contains the vital vitamin K. Blueberries are excellent sources of fiber and phytonutrients. Avocados are good sources of monounsaturated fats that lower bad cholesterol and improve heart health.

White meats. These are an excellent source of protein and fatty acids. Fish provide omega-3 fatty acids which improve heart health and stimulate muscle growth. Chicken is a great source of protein, and it promotes the growth of muscle cells.

Grains. They are excellent sources of protein and dietary fiber that will keep you full. Grains also help in improving heart health and normalizing blood pressure.

Eggs. Eggs are excellent sources of protein, and they tend to fill you up thus minimizing hunger levels.

Tubers. Foods such as potatoes and sweet potatoes are loaded with essential vitamins and carbohydrates.

Dairy. Dairy seems to reduce the risk of development of obesity and type 2 diabetes. Cheese and whole milk are excellent sources of protein and essential minerals that promote bone development.

Summary

When you go on a fast, your body increases the hunger levels in an attempt to pressure you to look for food. Staying without food for a long time causes the body to switch to fats as an alternative energy source. When the carbohydrates supplying energy to the brain are depleted, the liver produces ketone bodies to supply energy to the brain. The food you eat (and the portion) will impact your hunger levels during the fast. It is important to consume healthy foods during the eating window no matter how strong the temptation to stray is. Some of the worst foods that you can indulge in while fasting includes sugary drinks, junk foods, processed foods, white bread and cakes, alcohol, and seed oils. On the other hand, some of the best foods you can indulge in would be nuts, fruits and greens, white meat, grains, eggs, tubes, and dairy.

PART IV

Chapter 1: What is Inflammation Anyway?

Did you know that inflammation is actually a good thing as long as it is limited in duration? Inflammation is the body's natural response to infection or injury. As the immune system begins working, minor inflammation is evidenced by the five universal signs: redness, warmth, swelling, pain in the injured area and unable to function. When inflammation becomes excessive, it begins to work against the healthy cells erroneously, which can lead to disease and pain.

Most people are familiar with inflammation after an injury. For example, a ballet dancer loses her balance and sprains her ankle. She notices the injured limb swelling and turning red. Upon touching the skin, it is warm to touch and there is quite a bit of noticeable pain. Finally, the dancer is unable to complete her routine because she is unable to continue to use her ankle and must have assistance with walking. This is inflammation in its normal state. This is what inflammation is supposed to do. Unfortunately, it doesn't always function properly. That's when inflammation becomes a problem.

When the body's tissue experiences bad stimuli, it responds in a complicated fashion with several parts including pathogens, irritants, or damaged cells and inflammation. Inflammation is the protector of the group and gets the help of immune cells, molecular mediators, and blood vessels. Inflammation's job is to eradicate the original reason for cell injury, eliminate neurotic cells and tissues that were damaged by the cause of the stimuli and subsequent inflammatory process, and begin fixing the tissue.

Inflammation is categorized into 2 types: acute and chronic. Acute inflammation is what we mentioned before: the initial response of the body towards the damaging stimuli. It is achieved by plasma and leukocytes moving around more from the blood to the damaged tissues. Chronic inflammation is basically just prolonged inflammation. That is the inflammation that causes problems for the overall health of the person.

Chapter 2: Inflammation causes what?

As mentioned before, inflammation is the normal process in which the body creates and sends out white blood cells to cleanse and annihilate alien matter in the bloodstream. When constant stress from external conditions or dwelling on past stressful events for extended periods of time, the levels of c-reactive protein elevates and creates chronic inflammation.

Chronic inflammation is detrimental to the body and can be the cause or the agitator of many chronic health conditions and it affects all areas of the body. In the gut, inflammation can cause Inflammatory Bowel Disease (IBD) which comes in a couple forms: Ulcerative Colitis and Chron's Disease.

Inflammatory Bowel Disease is a broad term that describes the disorders that require chronic inflammation of the digestive tract and can be crippling and can have potentially deadly complications. *Ulcerative colitis* is the cause for chronic inflammation and ulcers in the innermost lining of the colon (large intestine) and rectum. *Chron's disease* is the inflammation of the lining of the digestive tract and it frequently spreads will into affected tissues. IBD symptoms are varied depending on the location and the severity of the inflammation and may range from mild to severe. Symptoms common to both Chron's disease and ulcerative colitis include:

- Diarrhea

- Unintended weight loss

- Abdominal cramping and pain

- Reduced appetite

- Blood in your stool

- Fever and fatigue

Probably the most commonly recognized area to be affected are the joints. Rheumatoid Arthritis (RA) is an ongoing inflammatory disorder of the joints. RA affects more than simply the joints. It can sometimes damage the skin, heart and blood vessels, eyes, and lungs. Rheumatoid arthritis causes painful swelling and the effects can, over time, cause bone to erode and joints to deform. Sadly, despite new types of medication greatly improving treatment options, severe cases of rheumatoid arthritis still cause major physical disabilities.

In the early stages of rheumatoid arthritis, it is the smaller joints that feel the effects. It generally starts in the joints that connect the fingers to the hand and the toes to the feet. Over time, the disease symptoms spread to the elbows, wrists, shoulders, ankles, knees, and shoulders. The majority of the time, the symptoms occur in the same joints on both sides of the body. The usual signs and symptoms of rheumatoid arthritis are:

- Fatigue, fever, weight loss

- Tender, warm, swollen joints

- Stiffness in the joints (usually worse after inactivity and in the mornings)

About 40% of RA sufferers will have signs and symptoms of non-joint structures being affected:

- Kidneys
- Eyes
- Blood Vessels
- Nerve Tissue
- Lungs
- Bone Marrow
- Heart
- Salivary glands

Rheumatoid arthritis symptoms are fluid and will come and go. Flare-ups, times when the disease is more active, alternate with times of brief relief from the symptoms. Long-term effects may cause joints to move out of place and become deformed.

Another area of the body that can be adversely affected by chronic inflammation is the heart. Myocarditis is the inflammation of the actual heart muscle (a.k.a. myocardium) and can affect not only the muscle itself but also its vitally important electrical system. If the electrical system goes haywire, then the heart is not as able to pump and the result is rapid or abnormal heart rhythms (a.k.a. arrhythmias). The usual culprit that causes myocarditis is a viral infection, but it has been known to be the result of a reaction to a medication or simply a very general inflammatory condition. Severe myocarditis is potentially very harmful to your overall health. It weakens the heart to the point that the remainder of the body is unable to receive adequate amounts of blood. Over time, clots can form in the heart that left unchecked could result in a stroke or heart attack.

Because of how serious the consequences of this inflammatory disease, it is of great importance to know the symptoms of myocarditis and to take action at the earliest signs. Mild cases or very early on, there may be no symptoms or mild ones—say, some chest pain or shortness of breath. On the more serious cases, the symptoms and signs do vary depending on the actual cause of the disease. Symptoms and telltale signs to watch for are:

- Shortness of breath (no matter if actively doing something or resting)
- Swelling of ankles, feet, or legs with fluid retention
- Chest pain
- Arrhythmias (abnormal or rapid heart rhythms)
- Fatigue
- Various other symptoms and signs conducive to a viral infection (a headache, body aches, sore throat, diarrhea, joint pain, or fever)

Children who develop myocarditis may have different distinct symptoms:

- Arrhythmias (abnormal or rapid heart rhythms)
- Breathing difficulties
- Rapid breathing

- Fainting

- Fever

Another common condition that gets attention is not readily acquainted with inflammation among the general population conversation. This surprise condition is psoriasis. The common skin condition accelerates the life cycle of skins, thus causing skin cells to quickly layer up on top of each other. The resulting additional skin cells form painful and itchy red scaly patches. Like other inflammatory conditions, psoriasis comes and goes often. While there is no current cure for the chronic condition, the main treatment goal is to slow the growth of skin cells. Lifestyle changes (managing stress, cease smoking, applying moisturizers) may help with the uncomfortable symptoms:

- Swollen and stiff joints

- Dry and cracking skin that may bleed

- Red patches of skin covered with thick silver-colored scales

- Soreness, burning, or itching

- Pitted, ridged, or thickened nails

- Small spots that scale (especially in children)

Majority of the types of psoriasis go through flare-up cycles that can be for weeks at a time to months in a row. The flare-ups may be followed by a period of easing up or even complete remission.

There are actually several different types of psoriasis including Plaque, Nail, Guttate, Inverse, Pustular Erythrodermic, and Psoriatic Arthritis. They cover just about every area of the body and each has their own set of symptoms and discomforts.

Although the scientific community is still researching, there have been some studies that suggest that inflammation has a role in cancer. Harvard University conducted a study in 2014 that suggested the risk of colorectal cancer was possibly higher if the body had inflammation. The results concluded that obese teenagers with high levels of inflammation had a 63% greater risk of developing colorectal cancer during adulthood. However, their many variables of the study subjects made it unrealistic to make a definite claim. The Mayo Clinic states that gene mutations that occur after birth are not inherited and can be caused by a number of possible outside forces including radiation, viruses, smoking, carcinogens, hormones, lack of exercise, obesity, and of course chronic inflammation.

Inflammation causes less serious negative effects as well such as sabotaging sleep. In 2009, Case Western Reserve University conducted a study in which people reported less or more sleep than average had elevated levels of inflammation-related proteins in their systems. Paradoxically, insufficient sleep can cause an increase of inflammation and fluid buildup.

Chronic inflammation is bad for the lungs as well. The results are infections, asthma and COPD (emphysema and chronic bronchitis). Both asthma and any version of COPD cause shortness of breath and limits the daily activities of a person resulting in a quality of life that may be less than desirable.

Periodontitis is an infection of gums. This is a seriously damaging condition. Damage is done to the soft tissue and the bone supporting your teeth gets destroyed. Periodontitis can loosen teeth or lead to absolute loss of teeth. The good news is this infection is very preventable and treatable. The initial treatment is a recommendation the person works on improving oral hygiene by brushing twice a day, daily flossing, and getting regular dental checkups. If the gums are firm and pale pink fitting snuggly around each tooth, they are indeed healthy. If the following symptoms are present, they are indicative of periodontitis and an exam and treatment by a dentist is highly recommended. Signs and symptoms to look for are:

- Painful chewing

- Bad breath

- Easy to bleed gums

- Tender-to-touch gums

- Swollen or puffy gums

- Bright red, purplish, or dusky red gums

- Gums that recede making your teeth to appear longer than normal

- Pus between teeth and gums

- Loose teeth

- Spaces developing between teeth and gums

- Changes in how your teeth fit when biting

Like Psoriasis, there are several typed of periodontitis with three being the most common: *Chronic, Aggressive,* and *Necrotizing periodontal disease.* Chronic periodontitis is the most common, caused by plaque buildup and has a slow deterioration that, over time, improves and worsens but will cause destruction if left untreated. Aggressive periodontitis onsets in childhood or early adulthood. It tends to be a hereditary trait causing quick disintegration of bone and loss of teeth if not treated. Necrotizing periodontal disease generally occurs in people with weakened immune systems (HIV, cancer, or other causes) and malnutrition.

Other problems associated with inflammatory conditions are bone damage and depression. The inflammation can prevent bone-building nutrients being absorbed such as calcium and vitamin D. Chronic inflammation can be linked to depression as well and is responsible for depressive symptoms such as low mood, poor sleep, and lack of appetite.

With all these negative effects of inflammation, it is important to understand what inflammation is, what conditions it causes or aggravates, and how to treat it. Once inflammation is understood, then steps can be taken to prevent, treat, or eliminate the chronic inflammation. One important step to take is making lasting lifestyle changes such as choosing an anti-inflammatory diet plan to follow.

Chapter 3: Which Diet plan Works for you?

So the inflammation is in there, now what? First and foremost, seeking and following the advice of your primary care physician is crucial to proper treatment. He or she is already familiar with your medical history and lifestyle. They can make recommendations that are custom-made for your situation. Most likely, the first recommendation of any physician will be mild to moderate lifestyle changes depending on the type and severity of the inflammation. The first step to take is changing up dietary behaviors. Thankfully, with the heightened awareness and celebrities trying every diet out there, the common population has several diet plans to choose from— many of which have anti-inflammatory tendencies.

Dr. Weil's Anti-Inflammatory Diet is currently one with some popularity. It is not a weight loss plan. However, it is possible and perhaps likely that some minimal weight loss can occur. It is rather a strategic plan for choosing and preparing foods that have anti-inflammatory properties. The selections are chosen based on scientific knowledge on how they can assist the body to maintain ideal health.

Dr. Andrew Weil, a Harvard medicine graduate, is a best-selling author, internal medicine instructor and the framer and director of the University of Arizona in Tucson's Program of Integrative Medicine (PIM), which he founded back in 1994. He informs and gives insight on how to use traditional and complementary medicine techniques to utilize fully the body's natural healing mechanics.

Dr. Weil's anti-inflammatory diet plan is based on a foundation of plant-based foods with a recommendation of eating 4-5 vegetables and 3-4 fruits a day. From there, he uses a pyramid formation for the distribution of other food categories. Unlike the USDA recommended food pyramid with only 6 sections, Weil's pyramid has 15 sections. The detailed pyramid may seem daunting at first, but if it is looked at as an illustration of the entire diet plan, then it becomes easier to understand.

Fruits and vegetables are the foundation of the plan. It is recommended to eat organic or local produce is chosen over imported. The next row is made up of up to 5 servings per day of whole or cracked grains, 3 servings per week of pasta, 2 servings per day of legumes and beans. Next are friendly fats: extra-virgin olive oil, nuts, avocados, and seeds (5-7 servings per day). The fourth row emphasizes consuming omega-3 rich fish and shellfish (2-6 times a week). The next row recommends 1-2 servings per day of tofu, edamame, and other whole soy products. Above that row are cooked Asian mushrooms. The benefits of the fungi must be phenomenal because the dieter is permitted to eat unlimited amounts of this one food type. Above them in smaller amounts are other sources of protein. Finally, the top 5 categories are: healthy herbs and spices (in unlimited amounts), tea (white or oolong, 2-4 cups per day), supplemental vitamins (daily), healthy sweets such as dark chocolate (very sparingly) and if any alcohol is consumed, it should be red wine with less than 1-2 glasses a day.

Dr. Weil's plan, although rather specific, is simple in idea. Basically, avoid all processed foods. Soda and junk food are filled with artificial flavors and colors, and the chemicals used to create them are oftentimes conducive to inflammation rather than reducing it. Look for his diet plan books online and at your favorite bookstore.

The Mediterranean diet (a.k.a. arthritis diet) is an excellent anti-inflammatory diet plan. Many physicians nowadays are recommending it to their arthritis patients. The Mediterranean diet allows minimal amounts of bad fats and non-organic foods while encouraging consuming an abundance of vegetables, fish, fruits, beans, as well as nuts. The diet receives praises for its anti-aging and disease-fighting abilities.

Possible outcomes after eating these foods could include:

- Curbing inflammation (easing arthritis)

- Protection against chronic conditions (cancer, stroke, and more)

- Potential weight loss (great for joint pain)

- Lower blood pressure

- Happier joints and heart

Most anti-inflammatory plans share similar food suggestions: fish, nuts and seeds, fruits and veggies, olive oil, beans, and whole grains. The recommendations are in line with the Arthritis Foundation.

In 2004, a study revealed that those who consumed the higher amounts of omega-3 had lower levels of interleukin-6 and C-reactive protein, both of which have been connected to inflammation. The sea offers a vast supply of cold-water fish. Taking 600–1,000 mg of fish oil supplements can reduce swelling, pain, joint stiffness, and tenderness.

Eating 1.5 ounces of nuts daily (approximately a handful) reduces your chances of dying from inflammatory illnesses more than those who ate fewer nuts. One possible reason why is because nuts contain vitamin B6 which helps reduce inflammatory markers.

For modern dieters, there are apps such as Noom. Noom assigns the users a personal registered dietician. Noom is free to download the basic features on both iTunes and Google Play Store. Apple iTunes has the IF Tracker app that helps users find anti-inflammatory foods and build a healthy anti-inflammatory diet. Its list of over 2,000 generic and brand name foods track calories, fat, protein, calcium, potassium, sodium, cholesterol, carbs, and fiber.

Chapter 4: Quick Recipes to try at home

Probably the fastest sabotage of any diet is time. In this extremely fast-paced world, we need to maximize our time, and having quick meal ideas is a great place to start. In this chapter are recipes that are great to eat to reduce inflammation yet not take up a ton of time.

Chickpea and Vegetable Coconut Curry

Feeds 4. Time to the table: 30 minutes.

Ingredients:

4 scallions, sliced thinly

¼ cup chopped fresh cilantro

Steamed rice (optional)

1 can (28oz) cooked chickpeas

1 ½ cup frozen peas

Salt and ground pepper

1 lime cut in half

1 small head cauliflower (bite sized pieces)

1 can (14 oz) coconut milk

1 thinly sliced red bell pepper

1 tsp coriander

2 tsp chili powder

1 Tbsp extra-virgin olive oil

1 Tbsp minced fresh ginger

3 Tbsp red curry paste

3 minced garlic cloves

1 thinly sliced red onion

Directions:

Step 1: Heat olive oil! Pour into a large pot heat over medium heat. Sauté the slices of bell pepper approximately 4–5 minutes. Stir in the garlic and ginger, continue sautéing.

Step 2: Next, add the bite-sized cauliflower and toss well. Stir in the chili powder, red curry paste, and coriander. Cook until the whole mixture is slightly dark (about 1 minute).

Step 3: Stir in the coconut milk and simmer over a medium-low heat. Cover the pot and continue simmering until the cauliflower is tender (approximately 8–10 minutes).

Step 4: Remove the lid and squeeze lime juice into the curry, stirring to combine well. Add the peas and chickpeas, season with pepper and salt, then bring the mixture back to a simmer.

Step 5: Serve with rice (optional) and garnish each portion with 1 tbsp cilantro and 1 tbsp scallions.

White Turkey Chili Avocado

Serves: 8

  1 diced avocado

  1 can white beans (15 oz.)

  1 can (15 oz.) kernel corn

  4 cups chicken broth

  1 lb. ground turkey

  2 tsp ground cumin

  1 tsp ground coriander

  Salt & Pepper

  2 Tbsp extra-virgin olive oil

  1 diced onion (large)

  Minced garlic cloves (4)

  1 tsp pepper (cayenne)

Directions:

Step 1: Heat olive oil! Place in a large pot and heat to medium heat. Toss in the onion, cook until the onion is tender and clear looking (approximately 6–8 minutes). Stir in the garlic and sauté about 1 more minute.

Step 2: Add the turkey meat and brown until fully cooked (about 5–7 minutes). Once it is fully cooked, add the cayenne, cumin, and coriander, and then add salt and pepper to taste. Cook the seasoned meat until the aroma teases your senses (about 1–2 minutes).

Step 3: Add the broth and simmer over medium heat. Turn down the heat to low and simmer 30 to 35 minutes.

Step 4: Stir in the beans and corn, simmer for 2–3 minutes.

Serve by ladling into your favorite bowls then top with 1–2 tablespoons avocado and serve immediately.

Chicken and Snap Pea Stir Fry

Serves: 4   Prep Time: Approximately 20 minutes

Ingredients

1 bunch of thinly sliced scallions

1 thinly sliced red bell pepper

1 ¼ cup thinly sliced, boneless, skinless chicken breast

2 minced garlic cloves

2 tbsp rice vinegar

2 tbsp Sriracha (optional)

2 tbsp (plus extra for topping) sesame seeds

2 ½ cups snap peas

3 tbsp soy sauce

3 tbsp (plus extra for topping) fresh chopped cilantro

Directions:

Step 1: Heat the oil in a large sauté pan using medium heat. Next, toss in the garlic with the scallions and continue cooking until just tender (approximately 1 minute). Add the snap peas and bell pepper to the mixture. Continue sautéing for 2 to 3 minutes until slightly tender.

Step 2: Place the sliced chicken breasts in the pan with the mixture and cook until fully cooked and golden in color and the vegetables are tender. (approximately 4–5 minutes)

Step 3: Once the chicken is fully cooked and the vegetables are completely tender, add the rice vinegar, Sriracha (optional), and sesame seeds then toss the mixture well to combine. Simmer for an additional 1–2 minutes.

Step 4: Stir in the cilantro and garnish with a sprinkle of sesame seeds and cilantro.

Serve immediately for best taste.

Greek Turkey Burgers with Tzatziki Sauce

Serves: 4

Ingredients

¼ tsp red pepper flakes

½ tsp dried oregano

½ fresh parsley chopped

¾ cup of bread crumbs

1 minced sweet onion

1 egg

1 Tbsp extra-virgin olive oil

ground turkey (approx. 1 lb)

Fresh ground pepper and salt

Tzatziki Sauce

¼ cup fresh parsley, chopped

½ cucumber diced

1 pinch of garlic powder

1 cup yogurt

1 tbsp extra-virgin olive oil

2 tbsp lemon juice

Salt and black pepper

Toppings

½ red onion, sliced

2 sliced tomatoes

4 whole-wheat hamburger buns

8 lettuce leaves

Directions

Step 1: Preheat the olive oil using a small skillet then add the minced onion. After 3–4 minutes, add the garlic and sauté for an additional minute. Set that mixture aside to permit it to cool.

Step 2: Combine in a medium bowl an egg, parsley, oregano, red-pepper flakes and ground turkey with the onion mixture. Add the bread crumbs to the bowl and then season with salt and pepper. Stir well.

Step 3: While waiting for the oven to preheat to 375F, divide the mixture into 4 equal patties. Generously apply non-stick cooking spray to a large oven-safe skillet pre-heat it with a medium-high heat.

Step 4: Cook the patties in the skillet until each is seared on both sides (approximately 4–5 minutes each side). Place the pan in the warm oven to complete the cooking of the burgers (approximately 15 to 17 minutes).

Step 5: While they are cooking, make the Tzatziki Sauce. In a medium bowl, combine the cucumber, olive oil lemon juice and garlic powder with the yogurt. Salt and pepper to your taste preference then mix in the parsley.

Step 6: Toast the buns if desired and then add each patty to the bottom bun. To the top, add ¼ cup of the tzatziki, 2 leaves of lettuce, 2 slices of tomato, then the top half of the bun. Serve immediately.